The
SEX SPIRAL

ENDORSEMENTS

The Sex Spiral offers a message of hope to those enslaved in internet pornography. In a day where we see so much sexual brokenness, this book outlines a healthy theology of sex. We are so thankful for Dustin's story and the freedom that many will experience by reading this timely and informative book.

—Dr. Archibald Hart and Dr. Sylvia Hart Frejd
Authors of *The Digital Invasion: How Technology is Shaping You and Your Relationships*

If you want to understand the way sexual sin robs your soul of hope and joy, and the pathway to full life in Jesus Christ, then *The Sex Spiral* is the book for you. Dustin is candid, concise, and caring in his writing on such a difficult topic. There is hope for living a life of sexual integrity in the midst of a sexually confused culture, and this book will help you navigate this tricky terrain.

—Jonathan Daugherty
Founder & Director of Be Broken Ministries
Author of *The Four Pillars of Purity, Grace-Based Recovery,* and more

Fighting the lure of pornography is exhausting for so many. *The Sex Spiral* holds a new approach to experiencing both forgiveness and freedom in Christ and finally severing the addictive hold of sexual temptation. Bravo to Dustin Daniels for sharing these realistic triggers for every man to follow.

—Shaunti Feldhahn
Social Researcher
Best-selling author of *For Women Only* and *Through a Man's Eyes*

We may know our position on pornography, but that hardly helps the person entangled in porn to free himself. What we need today are more tools—practical, clear, Biblically based—so the habitual porn user can learn what to do about the problem rather than hear yet another sermon on how serious the problem is. Dustin Daniels has contributed just such a tool. *The Sex Spiral* is both an eye opener and a challenge, and those in bondage to porn, as well as those who minister to them, will find answers and approaches here.

—Joe Dallas
Author of *The Game Plan, The Complete Christian Guide To Understanding Homosexuality, and more*

The Sex Spiral offers an effective balance of biblical truth and practical application of that truth to the real-life struggle of sexual sin. Dustin shares openly from his own journey toward freedom, serving as an encourager and trusted friend to you as you read. This is a compelling resource that I'm delighted to recommend to anyone battling sexual sin.

—Dr. Juli Slattery
Psychologist and President of Authentic Intimacy
Author of *Sex and the Single Girl* and *Pulling Back the Shades*

The SEX SPIRAL

Forgiven and Free From Pornography

DUSTIN DANIELS

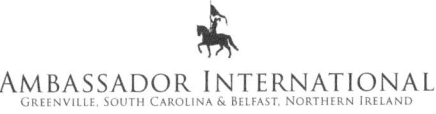

AMBASSADOR INTERNATIONAL
GREENVILLE, SOUTH CAROLINA & BELFAST, NORTHERN IRELAND

www.ambassador-international.com

The Sex Spiral
Forgiven and Free from Pornography
© 2018 by Dustin Daniels
All rights reserved

ISBN: 978-1-62020-607-2
eISBN: 978-1-62020-680-5

Unless otherwise indicated, Scriptures taken from the Holy Bible, New Living Translation, copyright © ©1996, 2004, 2007, 2013, 2015 by Tyndale House Foundation. Used by permission of Tyndale House Publishers Inc., Carol Stream, Illinois 60188. All rights reserved.

The ESV® Bible (The Holy Bible, English Standard Version®). ESV® Text Edition: 2016. Copyright © 2001 by Crossway, a publishing ministry of Good News Publishers. The ESV® text has been reproduced in cooperation with and by permission of Good News Publishers. Unauthorized reproduction of this publication is prohibited. All rights reserved.

The New Revised Standard Version Bible, copyright © 1989 the Division of Christian Education of the National Council of the Churches of Christ in the United States of America. Used by permission. All rights reserved.

THE HOLY BIBLE, NEW INTERNATIONAL VERSION®, NIV® Copyright © 1973, 1978, 1984, 2011 by Biblica, Inc.® Used by permission. All rights reserved worldwide.

Scripture taken from The Voice™. Copyright © 2008 by Ecclesia Bible Society. Used by permission. All rights reserved.

Scripture taken from The Message. Copyright © 1993, 1994, 1995, 1996, 2000, 2001, 2002. Used by permission of NavPress Publishing Group.

Cover Design by Sam Pagel & Mick McGinty
Typesetting by Hannah Nichols
Ebook Conversion by Anna Riebe Raats

AMBASSADOR INTERNATIONAL
Emerald House
411 University Ridge, Suite B14
Greenville, SC 29601, USA
www.ambassador-international.com

AMBASSADOR BOOKS
The Mount
2 Woodstock Link
Belfast, BT6 8DD, Northern Ireland, UK
www.ambassadormedia.co.uk

The colophon is a trademark of Ambassador

This book is dedicated to Jesus Christ, my Savior God.
Thank You for the gifts of forgiveness *and* freedom.

ACKNOWLEDGMENTS

This book would not be possible without the love and support of my wife, Amy. I love and adore you! Thank you for showing me what Biblical marriage is.

This book would also not be possible without Dr. Bruce McNicol and his team at TrueFace. Thank you for allowing me to use your "Control Cycle" material as the foundation for this book.

Special thanks to all of my mentors that poured your life into mine and my Brothers at Second Baptist Church in Houston that started this purity journey. Thank you for welcoming me, loving me, and pointing me to Jesus.

A very special thanks to Mark R. Miller, John Dooley, Troy Comstock, Greg Harman, Darien Bennett, Mike Turner, Jon Cline, Brad Edson, Jonathan Roe, Nick Ford, Susan Stacey, Doug Geist, Will Hopkins, Jay Flagg, Jason Lehman, Sam Pagel, Ben Tweedy, Dr. Dallas Bivins and Dr. Paul Smith. Thank you for pouring your life into me at God's appointed time.

Thanks to all the families of Seven Places Ministries. Thank you for teaching me more than I could ever teach you.

Extraordinary thanks to the team at Ambassador International: Tim Lowry, Sam Lowry, Katie Cruice Smith, Anna Raats, and Hannah Nichols. Thank you for trusting a nobody with a message that's for everybody.

CONTENTS

FOREWORD	13
INTRODUCTION	15
CHAPTER 1 AN OVERVIEW OF BIBLICAL SEXUALITY	31
CHAPTER 2 SEXUAL SIN	47
CHAPTER 3 TRIGGER #1: AWARENESS	57
CHAPTER 4 TRIGGER #2: SHAME	73
CHAPTER 5 TRIGGER #3: TEST / TEMPTATION	91
CHAPTER 6 TRIGGER #4: RESISTANCE	105
CHAPTER 7 TRIGGER #5: RATIONALIZATION	111
CHAPTER 8 TRIGGER #6: CONCEALMENT	123
CHAPTER 9 TRIGGER #7: ACTING OUT IN SIN	131
CHAPTER 10 TRIGGER #8: RELATIONAL WITHDRAW	141

CHAPTER 11
  TRIGGER #9: JUSTIFICATION   149

CHAPTER 12
  TRIGGER #10: BLAME   159

CHAPTER 13
  TRIGGER #11: ANGER   167

CHAPTER 14
  TRIGGER #12: HOPELESSNESS   177

CHAPTER 15
  THE ANSWER: LIVING IN FREEDOM   181

  EPILOGUE   197

  BIBLIOGRAPHY   199

  DISCOGRAPHY   205

FOREWORD

RECENTLY, A COLLEAGUE OF MINE wrote a very discouraging e-mail. He asked, "Mark are we losing the war?" By that he meant that there are many days when it seems like we Christian counselors are having no effect on our sexually-saturated culture. All of us who are old enough to remember the more innocent times of the 1950s have seen the explosive growth of pornography and sexually-explicit behaviors too numerous to mention. It does seem like Christians have lost the battle for the soul of our culture. My good friend Josh McDowell has called the current situation the greatest moral crisis in the history of the Church.

I wrote my colleague back and simply said that we are called to be a witness to the "remnant," those few who are Christ followers and seek a moral path. We are the minority. Our nation has lost its way. Great moral declines like this are familiar to the Church. The apostle Paul describes the moral decline that eventually led to the decline of the Roman Empire in the first chapter of his letter to the Romans. Later in that same letter Paul writes that we should not be conformed to the ways of the world, but be transformed by the transformation of our minds.

That is our challenge today. To be transformed by the renewing of our minds. We Christians are always called to be the "light" to the nations. We will be the minority. We therefore need voices of truth to constantly encourage us in this daily struggle. We will doubt ourselves and be challenged by the measures of Satan spoken through the voices of our culture. To tell the truth is often the unpopular and well-criticized path. It takes great courage.

I have known Dustin Daniels for quite some time now. He has been a "voice crying in the wilderness" or more accurately the desert of Arizona. His has been a strong and biblical voice over the airwaves of his radio show. He has spoken and taught the truth. Now he has put his wisdom in this book. I encourage you to read it and be blessed. My further encouragement is that you too will be part of the remnant who doesn't conform to culture. I encourage you to be a person of moral integrity. Finally, I hope that you will be a voice of truth to those you influence, perhaps mainly your own family.

—Mark Laaser, M.Div., PhD.

Dr. Laaser is nationally recognized as the leading authority in the field of sexual addiction and healthy sexuality with over 29 years of recovery experience. Mark has written fifteen books on the subject of sexual addiction.

INTRODUCTION

I WAS STANDING IN A closet with a loaded 9mm gun in my hand. I was hiding from an unexpected guest. I don't remember how long I was in there, but it seemed like forever. Regardless, I was somewhere I shouldn't have been—having relations with a woman who wasn't mine. Her son had decided to stop by and check on his mom. He had heard that she had moved out and was planning on filing for divorce. After he finally left, his mother opened the closet door to let me know it was "safe" to come out of hiding. She saw the gun in my hand, looked at me, and said with a scowl, "What were you going to do—shoot him?"

How does someone end up in that situation? I mean, this is the kind of stuff you watch on the local news. We think to ourselves, *This kind of stuff would never happen to me. What an idiot!* Well, idiot or not, up to this point in my life, most people would have told you that I was a really nice guy, a great employee, and a good neighbor. What they didn't know—what nobody knew—was that for over twenty years of my life, I was addicted to pornography.

I certainly didn't plan on becoming an addict, nor did I wake up one day and choose to become one. So how on earth did this happen? In other words, how does a child who found his father's collection of pornography wind up in a closet, hiding like a coward and still acting like that little boy—only now with a loaded gun in his hand—over twenty years later?

This book is somewhat of a narrative of how that happened to me, but more importantly, it's instructional. *The Sex Spiral* is saturated with God's Word and practical application to prevent the same idiotic type of thing from happening to you. Ultimately, this book isn't about me or you. It's about Jesus Christ and the grace He offers to sexual sinners through a blood-stained, Roman cross.

I find it fascinating that Jesus' first sermon came directly from Isaiah 61:1 (ESV): ***"The Spirit of the Lord God is upon me, because the Lord has anointed me (Jesus) to bring good news to the poor; he has sent me to bind up the brokenhearted, to proclaim liberty to the captives, and the opening of the prison to those who are bound."*** [1]

That passage is really, *really* good news. Read it again, this time slowly and out loud from the New Living Translation: ***"The Spirit of the Sovereign Lord is upon me, for the Lord has anointed me to bring good news to the poor. He has sent me to comfort the brokenhearted and to proclaim that captives will be released and prisoners will be freed."***

Are you beaten down and brokenhearted? Would you like to feel true comfort? Do you feel like a prisoner inside your own, self-imposed prison cell? Is the thought of being free from pornography only wishful thinking? Well, you're in good company, my friend, because you're not alone.

WE'RE DROWNING

When I was a child, my dad and I were playing on this pontoon-type raft at the lake. It had worn-out, sun-blazed, greenish blue, putting green carpet on the top. It was tied down by some sort of makeshift anchor. There were several teenagers playing on the raft as well. They soon began rocking the raft from side to side—up and down, up and down. I moved to the middle of the raft because I got scared and asked my dad, "Is it going to flip?" He reassured me that it wasn't. Needless to say, my dad was not a prophet; as those words exited his mouth, the whole raft tumbled over.

Everyone dove off, but I didn't know how to dive, let alone swim! I jumped as far as I could into the water, but the raft came crashing down

---

[1] *The Holy Bible: English Standard Version*. Wheaton: Standard Bible Society, 2016.

on me. I was in the water for just a nanosecond before it slammed onto my head, pushing me further underneath the water. I opened my eyes, and all I could see was that greenish blue carpet. I kept hitting my head on the raft, trying to escape, but it was directly over me. I was paralyzed with fear, and panic set in. I was gasping for air but only gulped lake water.

At this moment, I didn't need someone yelling from the shore, "Hey! You should have learned how to dive before you played on that raft." I didn't need another person pointing and laughing at me because I didn't know how to swim. I didn't need to be completely ignored, and I surely didn't need someone telling me to "try harder; just hold your breath for a little longer; and everything will be okay."

No, I needed someone to *save me*. I needed someone to get in the water, risk their own life, and pull me out from underneath the raft. I needed *someone else* to do something. My life was completely out of my control at that moment. Ultimately, I needed a savior. I was a little boy who was utterly helpless. I was drowning and moments away from dying. Thankfully, someone did save me. They grabbed my arm and pulled me out from underneath the raft. To this day, I still don't know who that person was.

Today, the Church is also drowning with its passive reluctance to address the painful reality of what's going on in our homes. Many people call pornography a "white elephant." I vehemently disagree. I believe we are way past cute metaphors that most people ignore. Lust is an enraged lion that is seething to devour Christian homes at a pace that human history has never experienced before. We have a pandemic of pornography in the pews of our Bible-believing churches that is destroying families while ferociously corrupting our children. Yet it seems that we have the same mentality for solutions—we're trying to give swimming lessons to those who are drowning.

For example, you know you need help with your porn problem, but the terror of telling someone (especially some type of pastor, minister or priest) has prevented you from doing so for years or even decades. You finally get the nerve to tell someone you believe is trustworthy, but, unfortunately, something like this takes place:

1. He immediately gives you a mental checklist of things that you "should" be doing and another checklist of things that you "shouldn't" be doing. Basically, he has given you more rules (laws) to follow.

2. He laughs nervously at the topic because sexuality is way too uncomfortable to do otherwise. He makes you feel like you're the only one with this "problem" and tells you to pray harder (whatever that means). He has essentially ignored you.

3. He spends enough time with you so that you can confess your sin. He also prays that God "will take away this desire," but, ultimately, there is no guidance, resolution, or plan as you walk out his door. He believes that he has done his part as a pastor and privately hopes that you will never bother him again. After all, he has a church to lead.

If one, all, or a variation of those things has happened to you, I'm so sorry. I truly am. I want to reconcile that conversation with this book, workbook, and video series.[2] I want you to know there are people who care and are willing to answer your questions on this journey toward sexual sobriety.

A BOLD STATEMENT

Christian evangelist Josh McDowell says that "pornography is the biggest threat to the cause of Christ in over 2,000 years."[3] Wow, that's a pretty bold statement, don't you think? Statistics are all over the board when it comes to how many men and women, boys and girls are viewing pornography—intentionally or by accident. Regardless of

---

2 Visit www.DustinDaniels.org to learn more.
3 *Dustin Daniels Radio Show.* "Let's Do Something About the Porn Epidemic." Episode 118. October 24, 2015.

what the stats are, my concern is that there are real people like you and your family behind those numbers. Those statistics represent people that are being raped by a lie. Ironic, isn't it? I could list dozens of statistics to prove why I think Josh is on to something. The problem with stats, however, is that those numbers won't change our behavior. If statistics actually had any influence on our lives, then we wouldn't smoke cigarettes, drink alcohol, or eat double cheeseburgers.[4]

"The Control Cycle"

I met Dr. Bruce McNicol of Trueface[5] in 2007. I read his book *TrueFaced* (now called *The Cure*[6]) and became an instant fan. I had the privilege of sharing the same office space with him and his team for more than a year. In that time, Bruce gave me an audio lesson titled, "The Control Cycle." I listened to it and was so excited about what he and Bill Thrall taught that I asked if he would be willing to modify it for sexual integrity, so I could teach it within the purity ministry of Seven Places®. He smiled and said, "No, but you sure can! It would be an honor for you to take our material and customize it." So with Bruce's blessing, that's what I've done.

Over the years, I've reworked and renamed this material *The Sex Spiral: Forgiven and Free From Pornography*. The reason for this specific title is because there are countless people sitting in our churches who are *forgiven* by the blood of Jesus Christ, but by no means are *free* to live the life God has promised them. Galatians 5:1 is prophetic: **"So Christ has truly set us free. Now make sure that you stay free, and don't get tied up again in slavery to the law."**

We have millions of people who go to church and raise their hands during the worship service on Sunday morning, yet they use those same hands to click on pornography only hours later. The Apostle James, the half-brother of Jesus, writes in James 3:10, **"And so blessing**

---
4 Smith, Bruce: Alliance Defending Freedom—Messaging University, 2014.
5 http://www.trueface.org.
6 Thrall, Bill; McNicol, Bruce; Lynch, John: *The Cure: What if God Isn't Who You Think He Is and Neither Are You?* Carol Stream: NavPress, 2011.

and cursing come pouring out of the same mouth. Surely, my brothers and sisters, this is not right!"

WHAT THIS BOOK IS AND IS NOT

Tragically, there are many Christian recovery programs that involve more psychology and human reasoning than biblical theology. This is heresy. We, as Christians, must first have a correct understanding of theology *and then* apply psychology and behavior based principles to our recovery. On the flip side, there are many colleagues of mine and many more faithful brothers and sisters in Christ who operate Christ-centered recovery programs. I would be remiss if I didn't acknowledge them here and thank them for being faithful to their calling in Christ Jesus.

With that being said, it seems to me that the most popular recovery methods of the past have lost their impact. It seems to be the same packaged and repackaged materials for different groups of people. I believe many recovery programs have never gained traction because they don't have the power to complete what they proclaim. The prophet Jeremiah writes in Jeremiah 17:14, **"O Lord, if you heal me, I will be truly healed; if you save me, I will be truly saved. My praises are for you alone!"** At the end of the day, most of us don't need ongoing and intensive counseling or therapy. We need discipleship that includes a correct theology of God's holy judgment on sin (Isaiah 6:1-8). We read in Proverbs 3:7b-8, **"... Fear the Lord and turn away from evil. It will be a healing to your flesh and refreshment to your bones (ESV)."**

Many programs rely on personal self-will and strength. Others focus on manmade rules that lead to more bondage. These things may change our behavior temporarily, but it will never set us completely free. Why? Because these programs refuse to get to the *eternal* root issue. Our biggest problem is *not* an addiction to pornography; it is a strained relationship with the Lord Jesus Christ.

Jeremiah writes again in Jeremiah 6:14-15, **"'They offer superficial treatments for my people's mortal wound. They give assurances of peace** *when there is no peace. Are they ashamed of their disgusting actions? Not at all—they don't even know how to blush! Therefore, they will lie among the slaughtered. They will be brought down when I punish them,' says the Lord."* Jeremiah also writes in Lamentations 2:13b, *". . . Your wound is as deep as the sea. Who can heal you?"*

The root issue in dealing with addiction and recovery is called *sin*. Therefore, *The Sex Spiral* specifically deals with sin. Its power comes from cooperating with the Spirit of God, engaging in the presence of God, and reading through the Word of God.

From a practical perspective, we will concentrate on *triggers*. A trigger is a thing or event that initiates the desire to engage in questionable behavior. A trigger could be anything—an attractive person, a picture on a magazine, a song on the radio, a certain aroma, a thought that crossed your mind, a good day at work, a bad day at work, a traffic jam, etc. It's important to know that a trigger is not a temptation or a sin, but it can certainly lead to that when not addressed immediately. Triggers explain the location as to where you are *right now* in the habit, bondage, or addiction to pornography.

Think of a trigger on a gun. When you pull the trigger back, something drastic is going to happen. You must make sure that your gun is pointed in the right direction, or someone will get hurt. Once the trigger has been pulled, a series of choices and consequences follow. These choices and consequences are two sides of the same coin. You can't have one without the other. Triggers are *immediate* feedback in your recovery journey, which then gives you an *immediate* course of action to exit your sex spiral.

The Sex Spiral is not a program like that of a twelve-step model, nor is it a Christian version of one. The twelve-step program is used as guiding principles that outline a course of action. These steps are meant to be long-range goals that members wish to accomplish. *The Sex Spiral*, on the other hand, focuses on the relationship and presence of the Holy Spirit through Jesus Christ as we learn our own triggers. So, rather than focusing on sin, we focus on our Savior. Think of it this way: steps in a twelve-step program are similar to looking at the face on your watch so that you can tell the time, while triggers are the little gears and motors underneath the face of the watch that show us how it operates. Triggers ultimately draw us closer to answering the question, **Why am I doing the very thing I don't want to do?** (Rom. 7:18-24).

The Sex Spiral will teach you God's design for sexuality, the triggers that lead to pornography addiction, and an exit strategy. This material can also stand on its own or be incorporated into any twelve-step program or purity group.

Make no doubt about it, pornography addiction is a series of predictable habits that we have created for ourselves. The bad news is that we don't realize it at first. The good news is that as you learn to cooperate with God by recognizing your own triggers, you (by God's grace) *will break free from the bondage of porn.* Jesus Christ did not die for your sin and rise from the dead for you to remain an addicted Christian!

With that being said, there is one last thing to consider as we start this journey together. I want you to consider letting go of everything you think you know about sex, addiction, psychology, pornography, recovery, etc. You have to give up trying to do this *your* way. Jesus gives us some insight into the recovery process in John 8:32, *"And you will know the truth, and the truth will set you free."* What Jesus didn't tell us is that the truth hurts like crazy at first. Many of us think we have the answers, but in reality, we don't even have the vocabulary to ask the right question. King Solomon writes in Proverbs 20:24, *"The Lord directs our steps, so why try to understand everything along the way?"* When we try to control our own recovery, we'll *never* get well. We are not in charge. God is. We are on His timetable. For you to become truly free from lust, you must lay down your ego by being silent and coming to the Lord as a child to be taught. The Prophet Habakkuk writes, *"But the Lord is in His holy Temple. Let all the earth be silent before Him"* (Hab. 2:20). Yes, indeed, true healing begins in the presence of a holy God.

Introduction

DEALING WITH ADDICTION

What does the Bible actually say about addiction? We see the English word translated only once in the English Standard Version in 1 Timothy 3:8: *"Deacons likewise must be dignified, not double-tongued, not addicted to much wine, not greedy for dishonest gain."* The Greek in the ESV literally means "to occupy oneself with, to devote yourself to." The New Revised Standard Version also translates the word *addiction* in Titus 1:7: *"For a bishop, as God's steward, must be blameless; he must not be arrogant or quick-tempered or addicted to wine or violent or greedy for gain."* The Greek in the NRSV is similar and translates the word *addiction* as "to give yourself over."

The Bible talks much more about being "a slave" or being "in bondage to sin," rather than "addiction." Why? Because the word *addiction* has a tone of victimization and hopelessness to it. In today's vocabulary, if I claim to be an addict, then it's really easy for me to blame others or circumstances. Therefore, I don't need to change; it's everyone else that needs to change around me. From a biblical worldview, this is unacceptable. The original Greek uses the word *doulos*, which means "slave." It's used 126 times in the New Testament. Unfortunately, its translation to English has been watered down considerably to the word *servant* or *bondservant*. *Doulos* is not only the idea of being a slave, but also the attitude that corresponds with being a slave as well. A slave is one who is completely controlled by someone or something.

The apostle Paul writes in Romans 6:16 (NRSV), *"Do you not know that if you present yourselves to anyone as obedient slaves, you are slaves of the one whom you obey, either of sin, which leads to death, or of obedience, which leads to righteousness?"*[7] It's important to notice the change in terminology here—moving from this concept of *addiction* to *slavery*. Whether we admit it or not, we spend time with the things or the people we love. In our context, a slave is submissive to impurity and controlled by wickedness. Jesus makes it clear in Matthew 6:24,

---

[7] *The Holy Bible: New Revised Standard Version*. Nashville: Thomas Nelson Publishers, 1989.

"No one can serve two masters. For you will hate one and love the other; you will be devoted to one and despise the other. You cannot serve both God and money." The word *master* means "lord" or "ruler." Jesus is talking about money in this context, but we could easily substitute the word "money" for "lust"—or any sin, for that matter.

CALLING IT WHAT IT IS

My personal healing journey toward sexual sobriety never included a twelve-step model, nor was it based in psychology. That's not a dig; it just is what it is. My journey included small groups of men at local Bible-believing churches with Jesus Christ as the foundation. In a word, it was *discipleship*. This is where I learned who Jesus is, who I am, and what sin is. These godly men called my perversion "sin" and *not* "addiction." If we want to learn how to walk in freedom from lust, we must call our behavior exactly what it is—*sin*. It's not a "mistake." We didn't "mess up" or "slip up." No, we willfully and consciously chose to *sin*.

2 Peter 2:19 (ESV) says, **"They promise them freedom, but they themselves are slaves of corruption. For whatever <u>overcomes</u> a person, to that he is enslaved"** (emphasis mine).[8] From this point forward, I will refrain from using the words "addict" or "addicted" but rather use the words "slave" or "bondage" instead as to be biblically accurate.

FACE TO FACE WITH A TORNADO

Being in bondage means that you are being held against your will. Proverbs 5:22 reads, **"An evil man is held captive by his own sins; they are ropes that catch and hold him."** When it comes to lust, we have created a habit, tried to stop, but ultimately can't. Maybe your behaviors have led to life-altering circumstances that are beyond your control. There's a good chance that your marriage, children, career and/or finances are being impacted as well. Regardless, you never intended your private porn use to impact your public life, but it has. That's why this book

---

8   *The Holy Bible: English Standard Version.* Wheaton: Standard Bible Society, 2016.

is called *The Sex Spiral*—because your involvement in pornography is destroying other aspects of your life—just like a tornado.

Do you know how a tornado works? A tornado is a violent, rotating column of air that usually develops from a thunderstorm. When moist air and cool, dry air collide, they create instability in the atmosphere. Tornadoes have windspeeds of 100 to 300 miles per hour, are anywhere from 250 feet to two miles wide, and can travel dozens of miles before they dissipate.[9]

Being involved with pornography is like personally inviting a tornado of unpredictable destruction and death into your life. When the reality of your life collides with your fantasy world of pornography, it's as if a tornado devastates everything you have ever known. It destroys everything in its path. Nothing is spared.

THE UNANSWERED QUESTION

So how does a little boy go from stumbling onto his dad's collection of pornography to winding up in a woman's closet with a loaded gun twenty years later? Are those two events even related? How in the world did some of my biggest life choices lead me down the path of two devastated marriages, bankruptcy, multiple career failures, dozens of ruined relationships, chronic depression, and suicidal thoughts?

The Apostle Paul writes in Romans 7:21-24, *"I have discovered this principle of life—that when I want to do what is right, I inevitably do what is wrong. I love God's law with all my heart. But there is another power within me that is at war with my mind. This power makes me a slave to the sin that is still within me. Oh, what a miserable person I am! Who will free me from this life that is dominated by sin and death?"*

---

9 Howard, Brian Clark. "How Tornadoes Form and Why They're So Unpredictable." *National Geographic*, May 11, 2015. http://news.nationalgeographic.com/2015/05/150511-tornadoes-storms-midwest-weather-science/, (accessed July 1, 2016).

I don't know about you, but it sounds to me like a sinner (dare I say "addict"?) wrote those words. It seems as if the apostle Paul somehow peered into my life. I was stuck in this spiral of desiring to do what is good but had no idea how to actually carry it out. At the end of my long, pathetic journey with lust, I felt like I had only two options for relief—more sex or commit suicide.

THE END GOAL

My goal in writing this book is to provide a biblically based purity plan that you can put into action the moment you are triggered. I will also answer the question posed by the apostle Paul in Romans 7:24b: ***"Who will free me from this life that is dominated by (sexual) sin and death?"*** (emphasis mine).

You've picked up this book because I'm guessing you've asked yourself a version of that same question. Maybe you're the spouse, parent, or friend of a loved one whose life is out of control because of pornography. Regardless, *The Sex Spiral* is a journey into the next chapter of your life. I actually like to call it a "beautiful disaster." Truly addressing your propensity toward lust is one of the hardest things you will ever do (as is coming alongside a loved one who is in bondage). Yet, it's glorious at the same time. Jesus said that we must learn to deny ourselves, take up our cross, and follow Him (Matt. 16:24-25). In other words, we must do what we don't want to do on a daily (sometimes hourly) basis.

This is why so many people start the journey toward sexual sobriety but never finish. They believe the lie that it's too painful to deal with the perversion that they've attached themselves to. It makes us sick to think of the secrets we're hiding. We find it nearly impossible to admit the depravity of our own hearts and to confess these evil thoughts that run through our minds. We underestimate the power of sin and overestimate pop psychology. Too much psychology empties the cross of its power. Being overly spiritual does the same thing.

Introduction

We also underestimate the name of Jesus Christ and overestimate our own self-will.

We fool ourselves into thinking that living a mediocre Christian life is good enough. After all, you've learned to function inside your dysfunction, right? We rationalize our behavior by saying, "It's just this one little part of my life. It's not that big of a deal. Nobody needs to know. I can take care of this myself." However, I'm living proof that God has so much more for you than an uninspired life, a mediocre marriage, and Facebook friendships. By God's grace in my own life, I will show you God's intentional purpose behind your sexual struggle.

I want you to know that I've struggled how to communicate this material in book form. I thought it would be fairly simplistic to take my teaching notes over the years and write this book. I thought wrong. The reality is that I'm used to teaching in front of small groups that provide immediate feedback and allow me to address questions and concerns on the spot. Obviously, that is not the case with this book. Unfortunately, you can't hear the tone of my voice or see my demeanor.

As I've written and edited this manuscript, I must confess that, at times, I found my words surprisingly blunt—especially in the chapters dealing with justification and blame. I've also struggled with using the personal pronoun "you." The last thing in the world I want you to think is that I'm angry with you and pointing my finger at you as you read. No, no, no. That's not my intention. My job is to confront your sexual sin, point you to Jesus Christ, and provide a biblical structure for you to walk this journey with Him. My intention is to come alongside you and teach you what the Lord—through others—has taught me. To do that, we must call sin what it is. That alone is a heavy pill to swallow (Rev 10:10). I will say some things that you won't want to hear, but please know that I say them in love—sometimes tough love. I will also share Scripture passages that will pierce your heart. This is where iron sharpens iron (Prov. 27:17). It is also where healing begins.

28 THE SEX SPIRAL

At the end of the day, you get to choose what you want to do with this information. So, with that disclaimer, I have chosen to use the personal pronoun "you" quite a bit in this manuscript. That decision makes this a very personal book. I actually was going to soften the book by using the words "I," "we," or "one." But, it was shortly after my decision that the Lord showed me Ezra 10:10, **"You have committed a terrible sin. By marrying pagan women, you have increased Israel's guilt"** (emphasis mine.) Yes, indeed my friend, our topic is not table talk. It's serious; and once we realize that, then we can move forward with solemn lamenting, reflective repenting, honest prayer, and sincere contemplation. This is where genuine change begins to happen!

THE ACTUAL SEX SPIRAL:

The Sex Spiral is a plan to experience not only the *forgiveness* of Jesus Christ, but also the *freedom* He promises—specifically from the sin of sexual lust. As you look at the spiral below, you'll notice that there

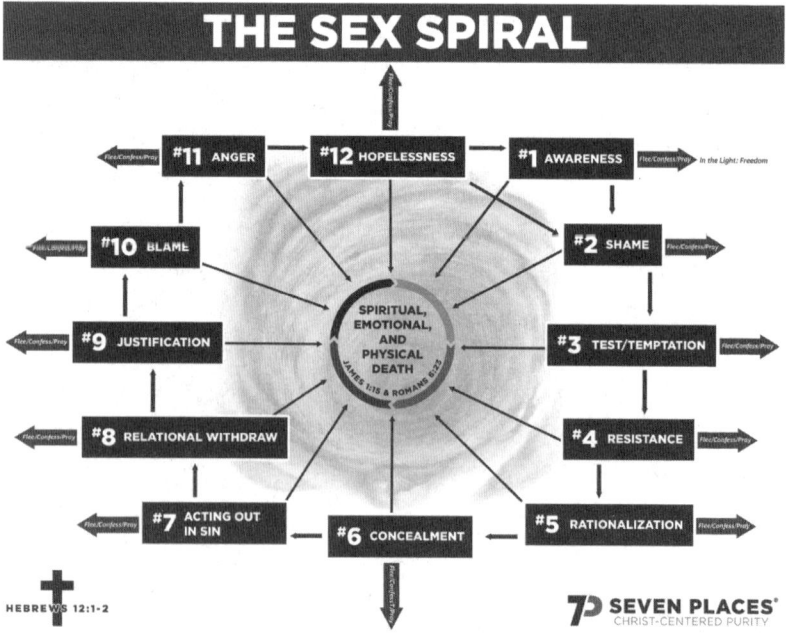

are twelve triggers. The rotation of these triggers is similar to that of a clock. We will spend a full chapter discussing each trigger in detail. You'll also notice that each trigger has an arrow pointing to a mini-spiral in the middle. The longer we stay in the spiral, the further we get away from God's presence. To exit *the sex spiral*, we have three choices:

1. Flee/Run
2. Confession
3. Prayer

You can flee, confess, and pray separately or in combination with one another. The goal of *The Sex Spiral* is to exit at the first trigger. As you start spinning around the spiral, it becomes increasingly harder to exit.

It's important to note that as you move through these triggers, it appears that you are spinning around in a linear cycle. In other words, it seems that we are starting at the same place each time. This is misleading because when we're involved with something as demonic as pornography, we never go around and start at the same place. Each time we start over, we move into a lower level of depravity. That's why when you turn this cycle on its side, it looks like a spiral or tornado.

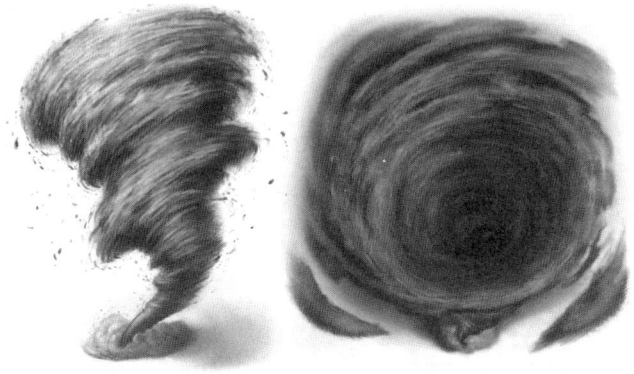

Before we dive into the actual triggers of *The Sex Spiral*, we first need context as to what sex really is, where it came from, and why we're so fascinated by it. Once we know what is right, we can then identify what is wrong.

CHAPTER 1

AN OVERVIEW OF BIBLICAL SEXUALITY

I WAS LYING IN MY bunk bed with a female babysitter. Turns out, we were both naked. I don't remember how old I was—maybe five or six. I'm guessing she was in her early teens. We had made a "fort" out of the bed earlier by hanging sheets and blankets from the top bunk. I don't remember exactly what all happened to me physically that day, but I do remember her pointing, laughing, and saying something about my body. I had no idea that her words would subconsciously control my life for the next two decades.

Several years later, I found my dad's collection of pornography in his spare bedroom. I still remember the way the room looked. It was small and simple, and it smelled old. I remember the wood paneling on the walls and where the bed and dresser were placed. Tragically, I also remember those pornographic photos, as they seem to be burned into the recesses of my mind. Those two events were my introduction to sexuality. So let me ask you this:

- Was this the right way to introduce a little boy to sex?
- What exactly is the right way?
- Who has the moral authority to determine the right way from the wrong way?

Before we move into *The Sex Spiral* material, I want to first discuss sexuality from God's perspective. Contrary to the sexual revolutionaries of our day, there is a right way and a wrong way to understand sexuality. Just as a builder uses a ruler as a fixed standard of measurement, a doctor uses a scale for our weight, and a banker uses math to calculate currency, God has also set a standard and a template for His children to abide by. Without God's moral standard on sexuality, we are left to our own individual opinions of what's right and what's wrong.

King Solomon writes in the Song of Songs 2:7 ***"not to awaken love until the time is right."*** Unfortunately, "love" was awakened way too soon in my life and possibly for you as well. And for that, I'm truly sorry. Those things were wrong. However, we can choose to start making those things right *today*. A big part of our healing journey is to renew our mind (Rom. 12:2) by learning what healthy sexuality really looks like from God's perspective. To do that, let's turn to the very beginning of human history and learn from our ancestors, Adam and Eve.

THE CREATOR OF SEX

I once had a woman tell me that Hugh Hefner, the founder of *Playboy Magazine*, "invented sex." I just stared at her in disbelief. Surely, she's kidding, right? Nope, she was dead serious.

As Christians, we recognize that God Himself is the Creator of all things—which, of course, includes sexuality. It's been said that God created man, and the devil slapped on our private parts. Many of us might not actually say this, but it seems that we believe it to a certain extent. For us to get the full picture of sexuality, we must start at the beginning. Unfortunately, many of us have heard the Creation story so many times that we've become numb to it. However, I would like to reintroduce it to you with fresh eyes and a soft heart. For us to truly understand what God intended with sex, we must first slow way down as we read from Genesis chapters one and two. It's also critically important to understand the meaning of the words in the original Hebrew language. With that being said, I'm going to teach you several Hebrew words which will give us a roadmap and provide much-needed clarity to learn God's design for sex, marriage, and the family.

An Overview of Biblical Sexuality

REVISTING GENESIS 1 AND 2

We read in Genesis 1:26a (ESV), *"Then God said, 'Let us make man in our image, after our likeness.'"*[10] Have you ever noticed that God changed His wording from the previous Scripture passages:

- *"Let there be light . . . "* (Gen. 1:3).
- *"Let there be an expanse . . . "* (Gen. 1:6).
- *"Let the waters . . . "* (Gen. 1:9).
- *"Let the earth sprout vegetation . . . "* (Gen. 1:11).
- *"Let there be lights . . . "* (Gen. 1:14).
- *"Let the waters swarm . . . "* (Gen. 1:20).
- *"Let the earth . . . "* (Gen. 1:24).

The words *let us make* in Genesis 1:26 mean "we will make man." This is where we learn that human life is created in the very image of God—"after our (God's) likeness." This is also the first time we see Father, Son, and Spirit working together as one. Now note here that although God says man is created in His own image, God doesn't tell us what the image actually is. A.W. Tozer says, "When the Scripture states that man was made in the image of God, we dare not add to that statement an idea from our own head and make it mean 'in the exact image.' To do so is to make man a replica of God. To think of creature and Creator as alike in essential being is to rob God of most of His attributes and reduce Him to the status of a creature."[11]

Secondly, notice the word *man* in Genesis 1:26. Contrary to popular belief, this is *not* a person named Adam! The word is ʾā·ḏām.[12] It actually means "mankind, humankind, and/or humanity." Therefore, this

---

10 *The Holy Bible: English Standard Version*. Wheaton: Standard Bible Society, 2016.
11 Tozer, A.W. *The Knowledge of the Holy*. New York: Harper One Publishers, 1961.
12 McDaniel, Chip. *The English-Hebrew Reverse Interlinear Old Testament English Standard Version*. Lexham Press, 2009.

verse could literally be read: *"Let us make ʾā·ḏām (mankind) in our image, after our likeness."*

Let's now replace the word *man* with *mankind* to give us a new perspective on this text, starting in Genesis 1:27 (ESV): **"So God created the** ʾā·ḏām (the man who represents all mankind) **in his own image, in the image of God he created him; male and female he created them."**[13] This verse could also be translated: **"He created people, both the man kind and the woman kind. In the image of God He created it**[14]**: male and female He created both**[15]**."**[16]

What exactly are the types of people that God created? From Scripture, we see that there are two:

1. Male—*zākār*. This Hebrew term simply means "being of the masculine sex." It specifically refers to a species that is *not* female. It also means "to remember." In other words, a man wants to be remembered for his legacy and accomplishments.

2. Woman—*nĕqēbâ*. This Hebrew word means "being of the feminine sex." The woman is the one that bears eggs or produces young. This word is a general term that specifically refers to *not* being male. It also means "hollow" or "hollow-spot"—referring to a woman's womb.

Obviously, these Hebrew words very much refer to the anatomy differences between male and female. Contrary to the world's confusion of someone being able to change their gender based on how they think or feel at the moment (gender fluidity), God is a God of order, structure, simplicity, and, most of all, reality. He specifically created only two versions of human beings (and of all species): male and female.

---

13 Ibid.
14 This pronoun is *hu*. *Hu* is translated as "he," "she," or "it."
15 This pronoun is *hem*. *Hem* is translated as "they" or "both."
16 Reyburn, W. D., and E.M. Fry. *A Handbook on Genesis*. New York: United Bible Societies, 1998. 51.

An Overview of Biblical Sexuality

DIGGING DEEPER

Genesis 1 gives us the overview of the Creation story and the impression that man and woman were created at the exact same time. Let's flip the page to Genesis 2 for the specifics and continue to apply our new understanding of the text by replacing the word *man* with *mankind*.

Genesis 2:7 (ESV) says, **"Then the Lord God formed the** ʾā·ḏām (the man who represents all mankind) **of dust from the ground and breathed into his nostrils the breath of life, and the** ʾā·ḏām **became a living creature."**[17]

The word *formed* in this verse describes the work of an artist. Could this be the reason that God changed His wording from *"Let there be"* to *"Let us make"* in Genesis 1? It's as if God also changed His tone here as well, don't you think? It seems as if He was slowing down and taking more care with this particular creation.

Secondly, let's look at the word *dust*. Dust can refer to ashes, debris, and rubbish. It's even defined as "crumbs of the earth." How much is dust worth? Nothing! People will certainly pay for dirt, mud, and clay when landscaping their yard, but not dust. Interesting, isn't it? To think that human beings are not just made from the ground, but specifically from the dust of the ground.

Speaking of the ground . . . the Hebrew word for ground is *adamah* (ʾăḏāmâ). Sound a little familiar? We just learned that the Hebrew word for man is ʾā·ḏām, which is a generic term for "mankind." Do you see the story God is starting to tell? From the ground, *adamah*, God creates *adam*, mankind.

Still with me? Let's keep going; this is where it gets really fun!

---

17 *The Holy Bible: English Standard Version.* Wheaton: Standard Bible Society, 2016.

36 THE SEX SPIRAL

Genesis 2:18 (ESV) says, *"Then the Lord God said, 'It is not good that the* ʾā·ḏām *should be alone; I will make him a helper fit for him.'"*[18]

Did you notice that this is the first time that God states that something is *not* good? Everything else was *very* good up to this point. It's here that we start to see the importance of relationships.

Genesis 2:21-22 (ESV) says, *"So the Lord God caused a deep sleep to fall upon the* ʾā·ḏām *and while he slept took one of his ribs and closed up its place with flesh. And the rib that the Lord God had taken from the* ʾā·ḏām *He made into a woman and brought her to the* ʾā·ḏām.*"*[19]

Let's now take a look at the word *rib*. Growing up, I've always understood it to simply be a single bone that was taken from a person named Adam. However, the Hebrew word for rib is *tsela* (ṣē·lāʿ).[20] *Tsela* comes from the words "rib, side, or side-chamber." Look at one side of your entire rib cage from your collarbone to your waist. This is your side-chamber. Is it possible that instead of God simply taking one single rib bone from ʾā·ḏām, God split ʾā·ḏām almost in half to create woman? I always pictured this as a very simple, clean, outpatient operation; but once again, is it possible that God cracked ʾā·ḏām wide open to create woman? Is it possible that God took a huge part of ʾā·ḏām that included flesh, bone, and, of course, blood? After this major operation, look what happens.

WEDDING BELLS ARE RINGING

Genesis 2:22 (ESV) reads, *"And the rib that the Lord God had taken from the* ʾā·ḏām *He made into a woman and brought her to the* ʾā·ḏām.*"*[21]

---

18 Ibid.
19 Ibid.
20 McDaniel, Chip. *The English-Hebrew Reverse Interlinear Old Testament English Standard Version.* Lexham Press, 2009.
21 *The Holy Bible: English Standard Version.* Wheaton: Standard Bible Society, 2016.

An Overview of Biblical Sexuality

The Lord is now *bringing* the woman to the man. This presumes that there must be some distance between the two, correct? Now, wait a minute, what does this look like to you? We have God (the Father) bringing a woman (His daughter) to be introduced to a man. Doesn't this resemble a father walking his daughter down an aisle to be given away to her husband? Of course it does! So how does ʾā·ḏām respond?

According to Genesis 2:23 (ESV), **"Then the** ʾā·ḏām **said, 'This at last is bone of my bones and flesh of my flesh; she shall be called Woman, because she was taken out of Man.'"**

Isn't it interesting that ʾā·ḏām admits that woman is not just bone, but flesh and, presumably, blood as well? Now, this is where it gets really interesting. Have you ever wondered why the words *Woman* and *Man* are capitalized (or italicized) in this verse?[22]

This Hebrew word for woman is ʾishshâh (pronounced *ish-shaw´*),[23] while this Hebrew word for man is *ish*[24] (pronounced *eesh*). Adam was consistently called ʾā·ḏām up until this point, but now something is very different. He's not the same. A large part of him is gone. It's in this verse that ʾā·ḏām no longer represents the entire human race, but, rather, God specifically creates two beings *from* ʾā·ḏām—man and woman. This is also where we see ʾā·ḏām representing mankind transition to *Adam*— a person using his proper name.

THE CREATION OF SEX

Genesis 2:24-25 (ESV) says, **"Therefore a man shall leave his father and his mother and hold fast to his wife, and they shall become one flesh. And the man and his wife were both naked and were not ashamed."**[25]

God now defines what sexuality is (and is not) in this verse. "Holding fast" is the concept of clinging together as one, to keep one

---

[22] These words may be capitalized, italicized, or in quotes, depending on the version of the Bible you have.
[23] McDaniel, Chip. *The English-Hebrew Reverse Interlinear Old Testament English Standard Version.* Lexham Press, 2009.
[24] Ibid.
[25] *The Holy Bible: English Standard Version.* Wheaton: Standard Bible Society, 2016.

another close in a very specific and strategic committed relationship that includes sex ("becoming one flesh"). Therefore, sex is the exclusive activity that defines the marriage relationship. It's the single activity that is reserved for husband and wife.

We can now see how God designed men and women. God split ʾā·ḏām in two, taking out the characteristics of femininity and leaving the characteristics of masculinity.[26] We must also notice that God didn't make an exact replica of ʾā·ḏām. Men and women are equals who are created by God to complement one another physically, emotionally, and spiritually. This is called *complementarity*. It means that men and women are equal *but different,* each having different roles and responsibilities in the marriage.

Ladies, did you notice that God created woman *last*? Is it possible that He wanted to make sure everything was just perfect with a home and husband before you were created? There is an old saying, "Save the best for last," but you have much more worth and dignity than a cliché. You are indeed a woman made in the very image of God—the pinnacle of God's creation!

Gentlemen, since women are the pinnacle of God's creation, could that be the reason that we are so intrigued by them? Could that be the reason we are drawn to their form and beauty? Is this the reason we want to be in their presence? Of course it is! When we look upon a woman, we see a glimpse of the beautiful holiness of God.

Question: What happens when husband and wife have sex— "become one flesh"? Are they not coming back together as one, representing ʾā·ḏām (mankind)?

They are. Now think about it. Does this explain the natural desire for companionship between men and women? Could it explain the sexual desire for men and women to come back together as one? I believe it does. Therefore, marriage is defined as:

---

26 Garlow, Jim, Blackstone Conference, Morning Devotion, Alliance Defending Freedom, 2013.

An Overview of Biblical Sexuality

Marriage: A lifelong blood covenant established by God between one biological man and one biological woman consummated (completed and fulfilled) with sexual intercourse (Gen. 2:24).

Why is marriage a *blood* covenant? Hidden in the female body lies a mystery that baffles biologists to this day. This mystery is called a hymen—a small lining of tissue that partially covers her vagina. When a woman has sex for the first time, her hymen is penetrated and causes her to bleed lightly.

Throughout the Bible, we read about God making a promise and then confirming that promise with the shedding of blood. For example, in Genesis chapters fifteen through seventeen, we read about God's promise to Abraham. The promise is to make him the father of many nations. Now, keep in mind, Abraham has no children and is ninety-nine years old when this promise is made. God makes this promise and also fulfills it—not only by the shedding of blood through animal sacrifice, but also by the circumcision of Abraham's foreskin. Thus, blood was used to fulfill *and* seal God's promise. The same can be said with God's covenant with King David that was ultimately fulfilled by Jesus Christ Himself.

Although secular biologists may not know what the hymen is for, I would propose that God specifically designed the hymen to fulfill *and* seal the marriage promise. Just as blood seals and bonds God's promises to His people, blood also seals and bonds husband and wife together in marriage. Blood is a physical manifestation of a spiritual reality that we'll discuss later. But for now, please note that *sex is what fulfills the spoken promises (vows) before God and man.*

It's worthy to note that marriage was ordained by God before any city was ever built, any nation ever formed, or any law ever penned.[27] Marriage is the first institution that God created. This inevitably tells us of its supreme importance. Marriage did not come from man and, therefore, cannot be redefined by man. When I refer to marriage, I'm

---

[27] Alliance Defending Freedom, Blackstone Legal Fellowship Conference, 2014.

referring to the biblical definition of marriage in Genesis 2:24. I'm not referring to "marriage" as defined by the United States Supreme Court in the *Obergefell v. Hodges* decision on June 26, 2015.

Humans are the *imago Dei*. We are created in God's image and reflect His beauty, glory, *and* sexuality (Gen. 1:26, 27; 5:1-2, 9:6). I know it's unusual to think about, but sex between a husband and wife actually brings glory to God (Song of Songs 1:1-4). God tells us to "be fruitful and multiply" (Gen. 1:28, 9:1,7, 26:4, 24, Lev. 26:9, Ps. 127:3-5). Therefore, sex reflects the creativity of God by a husband and wife becoming one, experiencing pleasure *together*, and having the capacity to create life *together*.

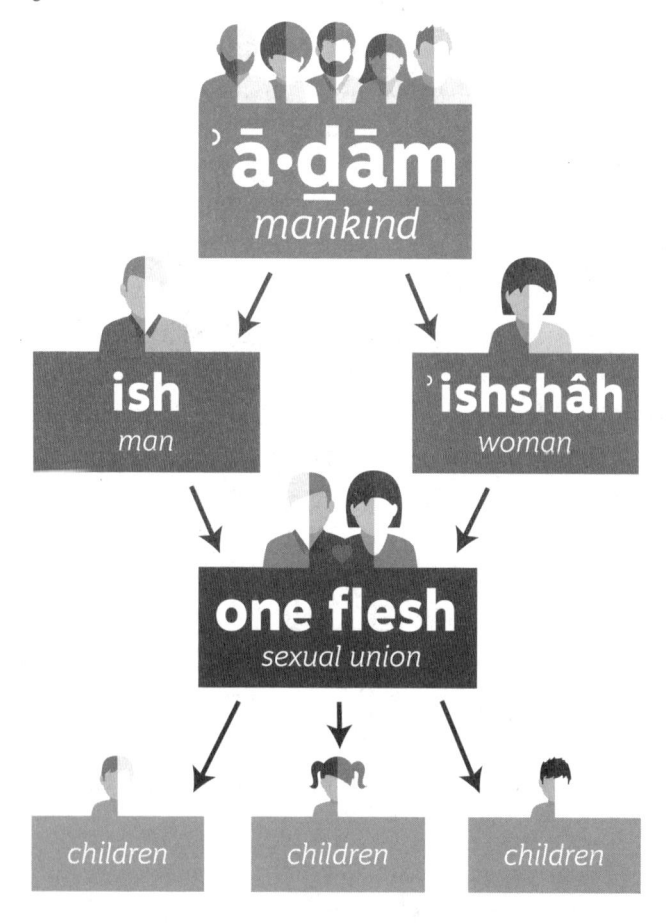

ʾā·ḏām
mankind

ish
man

ʾishshâh
woman

one flesh
sexual union

children   children   children

THE MYSTERY OF MARRIAGE

I've been married three times and divorced twice. I'm embarrassed and ashamed of my past. I'm a former liar and coward. My first marriage was out of ignorance, and my second was out of rebellion. To have to tell people my story and share my marriage failures repeatedly with strangers is humiliating to say the least, but that's the whole reason for this book. It's to show you what sex is and is not as defined by Almighty God Himself.

It's quite an understatement to say that my first two marriages were not what God had in mind. Undoubtedly, many people will call me a hypocrite to teach about sex and marriage from a biblical foundation when I've been divorced twice (which is fine, as I've been called much worse). Many people ask, "Doesn't God hate divorce?" As church people, we love to categorize sin, as if divorce and homosexuality are the only things that God condemns. Of course, God hates divorce. God hates *all sin*. In fact, He hates sin so much that God actually divorced Israel because of her adultery:

> **The Lord said to me in the days of King Josiah: "Have you seen what she did, that faithless one, Israel, how she went up on every high hill and under every green tree, and there played the whore? And I thought, 'After she has done all this she will return to Me,' but she did not return, and her treacherous sister Judah saw it. She saw that for all the adulteries of that faithless one, Israel, I had sent her away with a decree of divorce. Yet her treacherous sister Judah did not fear, but she too went and played the whore. Because she took her whoredom lightly, she polluted the land, committing adultery with stone and tree. Yet for all this her treacherous sister Judah did not return to me with her whole heart, but in pretense, declares the Lord"** (Jer. 3:6-10—ESV).

As we see in the above text, God has divorced us all because of our hard hearts. The good news, however, is that Jesus made everything right by proposing to us from a Roman, blood-stained cross (Lk. 23:34).

THE SPIRITUAL REALITIES OF MARRIAGE

Let's now transition from the physical side of sex and marriage to the spiritual. God also uses marriage as a spiritual illustration throughout the Bible. He calls marriage "a mystery."

> *For husbands, this means love your wives, just as Christ loved the church. He gave up his life for her to make her holy and clean, washed by the cleansing of God's word. He did this to present her to himself as a glorious church without a spot or wrinkle or any other blemish. Instead, she will be holy and without fault. In the same way, husbands ought to love their wives as they love their own bodies. For a man who loves his wife actually shows love for himself. No one hates his own body but feeds and cares for it, just as Christ cares for the church. And we are members of his body. As the scriptures say, "A man leaves his father and mother and is joined to his wife, and the two are united into one." <u>This is a great mystery, but it is an illustration of the way Christ and the church are one</u>* (Eph. 5:25-32—emphasis mine).

We are familiar with a man being called a husband and a woman his bride, but in this text, we see a great mystery unfolding. The apostle Paul is telling us that Jesus Christ is our Groom, and we, as His Church, are His bride.

Let me give you a really simple (and silly) illustration. Think of it this way: our earthly marriage is like playing baseball for the minor leagues. God is preparing us through testing, trials, and temptations for the major leagues. Ultimately, Christ's marriage to the Church is playing in the majors. Jesus sets the standard for all marriages. Why? Because Jesus Christ is the *perfect* Groom! He just happens to be married to an

An Overview of Biblical Sexuality

imperfect bride (that's us). Therefore, our physical marriages here on earth are much more important than we think. Marriage is teaching us a spiritual reality that we see in Revelation 19:6b-8: *"Praise the Lord! For the Lord our God, the Almighty, reigns. Let us be glad and rejoice, and let us give honor to him. For the time has come for the wedding feast of the Lamb, and his bride has prepared herself."*

In Genesis 2, God creates the institution of marriage; and in Revelation 19, Jesus Himself fulfills the covenant of marriage in His original design (Rev. 19:7-9). Think of these two marriages as bookends. God purposely weaves this theme of marriage throughout all of Scripture in between Genesis and Revelation. It's this picture that Jesus Christ is the perfect Husband while the Church (all believers) are His bride (Isa. 54:5; Hosea 2:19-20; Eph. 5:25, 32; Rev. 19:7-9, 21:9).

Ultimately, marriage is about intimacy. What makes marriage so special is the private, sexual union that is shared between a husband and wife. It's the idea of "knowing" one another intimately. Believe it or not, this is the kind of relationship Jesus wants with us and why He chose to use the analogy of marriage. I know it's a little strange to think of God in this way, so let me give you an example.

As we read God's Word, we learn God's eternal plan for marriage in Hosea 2:19-20, *"I will make you my wife forever, showing you righteousness and justice, unfailing love and compassion. I will be faithful to you and make you mine, and you will finally know me as the Lord."*

This word "know" in Hebrew is yādaʻ. It's the idea that we develop a relationship *through experience.* Essentially, we *become* known. It's the same word that's used in Genesis 4:1a: *"Now Adam knew Eve his wife, and she conceived and bore Cain."*

Yādaʻ is also found five times in Psalm 139:

1. *"O LORD, You have searched me and <u>known</u> [me]"* (v. 1 ESV).
2. *"You <u>know</u> when I sit down and when I rise up; You understand my thoughts from afar"* (v. 2 ESV).

3. *"Even before a word is on my tongue, behold, O LORD, You <u>know</u> it altogether"* (v. 4 ESV).
4. *"Thank you for making me so wonderfully complex! Your workmanship is marvelous—how well I <u>know</u> it"* (v. 14).
5. *"Search me, O God, and <u>know</u> my heart; test me and know my anxious thoughts"* (v. 23).

Hmmm, that's kind of weird. Those Scripture passages don't seem to be talking about sex at all. What's going on? Yādaʻ is the idea that we *become* known—to be clearly understood, cared for, chosen. It's to be known emotionally and spiritually—not just physically.

MARRIAGE VS. THE *ILLUSION* OF MARRIAGE

In the historic, biblical, Hebrew culture, many marriages were prearranged. A woman could be married around the age of puberty, while the man was generally slightly older.

Today, living in the United States of America, we can't even fathom such an event. Our culture is repulsed by the thought. So how is it possible that two people who didn't choose to be with one another can actually live with one another, work together, love one another, raise a family together, and thrive?

There's a difference between biblical marriage and worldly marriage. Marriage, first and foremost, is not about sex—it's about God. Unfortunately, we have allowed emotional sex to become the foundation of our dating and, then, marriage relationship. This has drastic implications on the health of the marriage as we see this in our divorce rates. Is it a coincidence that nearly fifty percent of high school students are sexually active,[28] while the divorce rate is steady at fifty percent? Of course not. We have allowed our feelings and emotions to rule our lives. The problem with *emotional sex* is that it's extremely volatile. We tend to believe that the better the sex, the better the marriage. This

---

28 Conklin, Kurt. "Adolescent Sexual Behavior: Demographics." AdvocatesforYouth.com. http://www.advocatesforyouth.org/publications/publications-a-z/413-adolescent-sexual-behavior-i-demographics (accessed August 9, 2017).

An Overview of Biblical Sexuality

couldn't be further from the truth. The pleasure of sex in our marriage doesn't cook dinner, pay the bills, or assist in raising children.

Real marriage—biblical marriage—is intended to *change us* into the likeness of Jesus Christ—the Groom of all grooms. It's through the covenantal relationship of marriage that we find true joy, not just temporary happiness based on emotional sex. This means that when marriage gets tough, we are to work out those issues as mature adults being husband and wife. We are to develop our communication skills with our spouse and sacrificially give to the marriage rather than quitting like cowards. **"God so loved the world that he gave his Son"** (Jn. 3:16—ESV).[29] Once again, my life is "Exhibit A," as I'm speaking from painful experience here. Sex *by itself* doesn't make a marriage strong. It simply adds to the overall emotional, spiritual, and physical health between husband and wife.

The reason that prearranged, Hebrew marriages worked was because God intended that we find romance *in and through marriage*, not before it and not outside of it. Did these Hebrew marriages work perfectly? Of course not! Everything is stained with sin (Gen. 3). We don't have to look much further than Abraham and Sarah (Gen. 16:1-2). Yet, even through all our sexual sin and the relational sin that has come from our decisions, God continues to move His plan forward, despite our rebellion. It's like God is the ultimate chess player. Yes, indeed, God is fundamental to marriage and manifested through this covenant between a husband and wife, witnessed by God in vows such as these:

to have and to hold

from this day forward,

for better, for worse,

for richer, for poorer,

in sickness and in health,

to love and to cherish,

until death do us part.

---

29 *The Holy Bible: English Standard Version.* Wheaton: Standard Bible Society, 2016.

Now that we know that marriage and sexuality were designed by God to be two sides of the same coin, let's turn our attention to what sex looks like outside the covenant of marriage. This is called *sexual sin*.

CHAPTER 2

SEXUAL SIN

I REALLY WANTED TO WALK out of my house and go to church, but I didn't know how. I debated on whether I should go week after week. Deep down, I knew there was a God. I was also convinced that He was mad at me because of the life I'd been living—especially since I had left religion behind when I went to college. Even during those college days, however, I just knew there had to be a God no matter how much I denied or ignored Him. I also knew that if I didn't do something different with my life, things would only get worse. I once heard someone say that if you don't want to hit rock bottom, quit digging! Unfortunately, it seemed that I had many layers to get to my rock bottom, and digging was apparently the only thing I was good at doing during that time.

After my second divorce, I had to figure out how to change my life. Church seemed like a good idea, but how does someone go to church if they have not been invited? Should I just show up and crash the party? I didn't know anybody, and I didn't know the rules because I hadn't been to church in years. I finally decided to go to a Christmas Eve service. I walked in and immediately sat in the very back row. I couldn't help but notice how happy everybody appeared to be. Everyone seemed to have lots of friends with perfect families. My soul immediately began to ache with jealousy.

It was during this time that I lost everything . . . again. My second marriage lasted five months. It ended in domestic violence when she assaulted me and landed herself in jail. I was lonely, broke, jobless, and suicidal. I thought to myself, *What am I doing in church? This is ridiculous.*

THE SEX SPIRAL

I don't belong here. These people don't get it. They don't get me. Why don't I just go home, drink a beer, and watch porn?

The church was pretty crowded, so I figured all those people were there for a reason. I talked myself into staying. I tried to act normal (whatever that means), but it was during the sermon that something strange began to happen. It was like I saw all of those perfect, happy families, and I wanted that. I longed for some kind of stability and joy in my life. I wanted something that those people seemed to have.

The pastor was about halfway through his sermon when I started to get emotional, but I didn't know why. I felt this overwhelming sense of emptiness and started to cry. I tried to control my emotions at first, but the more I tried, the more uncontrollable I became. Sadness hit me like a freight train. My crying became so loud and "unchurch-like" that the people sitting next to me started to move away. Oh, the irony. I was frozen in that pew just weeping an ugly, loud, deep, soulful cry.

Finally, when the sermon was over and the choir started to sing, I was able to compose myself for just a second before I bolted out of there. I went home and thought to myself, *What was that all about? What is wrong with me? And, by the way, how could God ever love me? The only reason that the pastor said that is because he doesn't know me, and he doesn't know what I've done. How could God possibly forgive someone like me—a pervert enslaved to pornography?*

What I didn't realize back then was that God doesn't love perfect people. His love is for *sinners*, and there was no doubt that I was one. But what exactly is sin—especially sexual sin? And why was it keeping me from going to church?

THE BLAME GAME

Let's pretend that this is your first day at church. You tell me that you've never been before, and you've never read the Bible. I then give you an assignment. It's to read Genesis chapters one through four, and then we would discuss it next week. What I didn't tell you is that

Sexual Sin

I ripped Genesis chapter three out of the Bible I gave you. Now, what kind of questions would you have for me the following week? Would you ask me, "What happened? I must have missed something because one moment Adam and Eve were in this perfect relationship with God, and the next moment their kids are killing one another. What did I miss?"

John MacArthur said, "If we don't understand Genesis 3, we won't understand the rest of the Bible. We cannot understand the solution to the problem, unless we understand the problem. We cannot understand the cure unless we understand the diagnosis."[30]

ADAM AND EVE HID

*"When the cool evening breezes were blowing, the man and his wife heard the L*ORD *God walking about in the garden. So they hid from the Lord God among the trees"* (Gen. 3:8).

I believe Genesis 3:8 is one of the saddest verses in all of Scripture. Adam and Eve *hid*. They tried to withdraw themselves from the presence of God. They tried to physically conceal themselves with itchy fig leaves from a tree. They wanted to be left alone. They ran from the sunlight into the darkness. They wanted to keep their actions a secret. Why? They knew they were naked and, because of their nakedness, they felt shame. Their shame forced them into hiding.

But, of course, they hid, right? They willfully and consciously rebelled against God's command. They did the *one* thing that they were not supposed to do. Wouldn't you hide?

This willful and conscious choice to eat from the tree that God specifically told them not to eat from is called *sin*. By its simplest definition, sin is rebellion. Adam and Eve's first sin didn't come from the eating of the fruit. It actually came before that. Their sin came from

---

[30] MacArthur, John. "The Fall of Man Parts 1-2." GracetoYou.org. https://www.gty.org/library/sermons-library/90-238/the-fall-of-man-part-1, https://www.gty.org/library/sermons-library/90-239/the-fall-of-man-part-2 (accessed October 2010).

their personal *decision* to rebel against God. Once *that* decision was made, it was only then that their behavior followed.

Due to Adam's sin, human beings are now born rebellious (Ps. 51:5). His sin has been passed down to all of mankind. This is called *inherited sin, original sin,* or *ancestral sin* (Rom. 5:12). The easiest way for us to understand this kind of rebellion is to simply hang out in a room full of children. My office used to be next to a preschool. One day I was walking to my truck and heard this from the playground: "JOHNNY, don't even think it!" About two seconds later, I heard a little girl start crying. Evidently, Johnny hit this little girl specifically *after* he was told not to. Why? Did someone teach him that? No. Johnny hit the girl because of *inherited sin*. He rebelled, just like you and I. We don't like to be told what to do. We don't have to teach children how to be rebellious; they just are. We are born morally corrupt because of Adam's original sin.

Secondly, there is *personal sin*. If we are born rebellious because of inherited sin, then we will make choices in rebellion against God through personal sin. Sin not only includes behavior such as lying, stealing, and adultery (see the Ten Commandments in Exodus 20:1-17), but it also includes attitudes and motives that are hostile and inconsistent to the attitudes and motives God requires of us (Gal. 5:22-25).

To understand personal sin, we must ask the question: What is my internal attitude, my motivation, my agenda, and my desire for choosing certain behaviors? It's critically important to understand that sin is not just my *behavior* but also my *attitude* that contributed to my behavior. Sin has the most serious of all eternal consequences. Each human being has a sin debt that must be paid. If the debt is not paid in this life by accepting Jesus Christ as Lord and Savior, the debt will be paid in the next life through eternal solitude and punishment (Rom. 6:23, Jas 1:15, Matt 8:12; 13:42).

I looked at Adam's story and realized how much hiding I had also done as a sexual sinner. After all, I not only physically hid from God, but I also hid my thoughts and fantasies—all in an effort to protect myself. The problem with self-protection is that it prevented me from finding the answer I was desperately searching for. I thought I was protecting myself by being alone, but the reality is that my isolation caused depression, depression caused hopelessness, and hopelessness eventually caused suicidal thoughts. I ultimately created my own self-imposed porn prison in my mind.

SATAN'S PERSPECTIVE

Before we discuss specific types of sexual sin, let's consider marriage from Satan's perspective. If Satan hates Jesus Christ (Isa. 14:12-15), and marriage represents the relationship between Christ and His people (Eph. 5:32), wouldn't it make sense that Satan would do everything he could to destroy earthly marriages and *promote* sexual sin?

I think it's imperative to note that the marriage debate, the porn pandemic, the divorce rate, gender identity issues, and the gay pride movement are all a battle that the Church must engage in from a spiritual perspective (Eph. 6:11-12, Dan. 10:10-14). The apostle Paul writes in Ephesians 6:12: **"For we are not fighting against flesh-and-blood enemies, but against evil rulers and authorities of the unseen world, against mighty powers in this dark world, and against evil spirits in the heavenly places."**

Sexuality is *the* spiritual battle of our current generation. Our enemies are not the pornographers nor the LGBT (Lesbian, Gay, Bisexual, and Transgender) advocates. Our enemy is the demonic forces that rule and rage against anything holy in this world (1 Pet. 5:8). In 2 Corinthians 4:4, the apostle Paul writes: **"Satan, who is the god of this world, has blinded the minds of those who don't believe. They are unable to see the glorious light of the Good News. They don't understand this message about the glory of Christ, who is the exact likeness of God."**

WHAT EXACTLY IS SEXUAL SIN?

One of the most popular questions to the Church is whether or not a certain sexual behavior is a sin. This sort of thing even happened to

Jesus. Religious leaders of the day were trying to trick Him regarding a question about divorce. We read about it in Matthew 19:4-6: *"'Haven't you read the scriptures?' Jesus replied. 'They record that from the beginning God made them male and female.' And He said, 'This explains why a man leaves his father and mother and is joined to his wife, and the two are united into one. Since they are no longer two but one, <u>let no one split apart what God has joined together</u>'"* (emphasis mine).

Instead of simply answering a question about divorce, Jesus answers their question by making a blanket statement about *all* sexuality. He points them back to Genesis 2:24. Jesus is telling us that ultimately no one or no thing should ever interfere with the sexual relations between one man and one woman in marriage. Jesus continues to answer their question in Matthew 19:8: *"Moses permitted divorce only as a concession to your hard hearts, but it was not what God had originally intended."*

God intended that we would love like He loves us—a loyal and sacrificial love that propels us to action for the good of others. Ultimately, we have strayed from God's original design for sexuality because of our "hard-hearts" (in other words—rebellion). Just as Moses gave the Israelites a concession for divorce, the Supreme Court has given full legal protection to homosexuality.

When people ask me if I *think* homosexuality is a sin, I tell them that it doesn't matter what *I* think; it only matters what *God says*. My response is to then ask them if homosexuality fits into God's definition of marriage as defined in Genesis 2:24. If it doesn't, then yes, God calls this sin.

We must think of Genesis 2:24 as a template, so the same rule applies to heterosexual sin like fornication, adultery, and masturbation. Do these behaviors fit inside God's definition of marriage as defined in Genesis 2:24? If not, then yes, God calls *all* these behaviors sin.

DEFINING SEXUAL SIN

We have learned that Jesus Christ is the perfect Groom. He is the *Groom of all grooms*. Jesus is our example in marriage and sexuality.

Sexual Sin

Therefore, when we talk about sex outside the covenant of marriage, we must take into consideration the biblical view on sexual sin. When it comes to the theology of sexual sin—to study the nature of God through the lens of sexual purity—we must define the actual behavior and then look at the behavior from a spiritual perspective.

Below are definitions of sexual sin, along with the *biblical view*.[31] This is not an exhaustive list but rather shows how these behaviors stray from God's original design for sexuality.

Adultery: Sexual intercourse between a married person and someone who is not his/her spouse.

Biblical View: Adultery miscommunicates that Christ will cheat on the Church and be intimate with another (Ex. 20:14, Lev. 20:10, Matt. 19:18).

Divorce: The legal dismissal of a marriage.

Biblical View: Divorce miscommunicates that Christ and the Church would be split apart after a certain period of time (Matt. 19:4-6).

Fornication: Sexual intercourse between two unmarried people.

Biblical View: Fornication miscommunicates that Christ and the Church experience sexual intimacy without commitment (Eph. 5:3, 1 Thess. 4:3).

Homosexuality (Sodomy and Lesbianism): Engaging in sexual behavior with someone of the same sex.

Biblical View: Homosexuality miscommunicates that the proper coupling God intended was not Christ and the Church (a man and a woman) but two "Christs" (a man and a man) or two "Churches" (a woman and a woman) (Lev. 18:22, Rom. 1:26-27).

---

[31] Lorence, Jordan, "The Vast Future of Marriage with Dignity," Alliance Defending Freedom: Academy Presentation. August 1, 2014, Laguna, CA.

The Church has sinned greatly in this area of explanation and care regarding homosexuality and same-sex attraction. We, as the Church, need to repent from our own pride and self-righteousness in this area. Jesus treated sexual sinners very differently than the church does today. He treated them with the utmost dignity and respect. (Jn. 4:1-43, 8:1-11). The subject of homosexuality seems to have two distinct categories. 1) People who are actively engaging in the physical, sexual behavior with someone of the same sex 2) The gay rights activists. The activists are demanding their rights as equal members of society.

It's imperative for church leaders to understand that inside these categories are people and communities of people who are as diverse as your church. For example, some homosexuals put bumper stickers on their cars, and some just want to be left alone. We must repent of our sin that generalizes all people into one particular group and instead treat each person as a human being made in the image of God, just as Jesus did.

Same-sex attraction, on the other hand, is not behavior but is, instead, the sexual attraction, interest, or desire for someone of the same sex. Attraction is not a sin; however, it can lead to sin through lust, fantasy, and behavior just as heterosexual attraction can lead to adultery and fornication. Unfortunately, the majority of the Church seems to lump everyone dealing with same-sex attraction into the gay rights activists category. This is a grave mistake on the church's end and is a sin to which we need to repent and ask for their forgiveness.

Masturbation: The stimulation of genitals to the point of orgasm.

Biblical View: Masturbation miscommunicates that Christ finds fulfillment with self rather than in exclusive devotion to His Bride (Song of Songs 1:1-4, 3:1-4, 4:12, 7:10).

Polygamy: The practice of having more than one spouse at the same time.

Biblical View: Polygamy miscommunicates that Christ has many churches, rather than one Church (Gen. 2:24, Matt. 19:4-5). Please note that I'm not referring to denominations.

Sexual Sin

Pornography: The emotional, spiritual, and physical abuse of people performing profane acts of sexuality for the arousal of a viewer or audience. Porn divorces the dignity of the person made in the image of God from his/her sexuality.[32]

> *Biblical View:* Pornography miscommunicates that Jesus Christ would derive pleasure from viewing such profane acts.

Prostitution: The practice or occupation of someone who engages in sexual activity for payment.

> *Biblical View:* Prostitution miscommunicates that Christ and the Church are strangers who experience a brief form of sexual union based on a financial transaction (Lev. 19:29, Prov. 23:27).

Rape: The crime of forcing another person to have sexual intercourse against their will.

> *Biblical View:* Rape miscommunicates that Christ would force Himself on an unwilling Church (Deut. 22:25-27).

Terminology

I would like to introduce some terminology that will be helpful as we move throughout the rest of this book:

Love: A loyalty and fidelity that propels us to action for the good of others—no matter the cost to me.

Lust: Experiencing pleasure without love; the moment we separate someone's sexuality from his or her personhood. God purposed us to have sex with a person (our spouse)—not a body.

---

32 West, Christopher. Difference between "nakedness without shame" and "shameless nakedness." https://www.youtube.com/watch?v=T1kHoAg4pxo&t=23s.

Sexual Sin: Any sexual thoughts, fantasies, or relations with someone or something outside the marriage covenant between one biological man and one biological woman as defined in Genesis 2:24 and Matthew 5:28.

Spiritual Strongholds / Spiritual Foothold: When sin is allowed in a person's thought life and moral belief structure and then clings to every facet of the person's life. This creates a pattern of faulty thinking based on lies and deception, which ultimately oppose God's truth (2 Cor. 10:3-6).

Picture a military camp with armed men walking up and down the concrete walls, fully armed and ready for battle. These men and all their defense systems are to protect what's inside the camp itself—the headquarters. This is where important decisions are made to protect the country. Inside the camp, however, the enemy has worked a stronghold. The enemy found a weakness in one of the commanding officers—a propensity toward pornography. So the enemy sent the officer an email with several pornographic images attached. Once he clicked on the pornographic image, it also launched a virus. This gave the enemy access to not only his laptop but also the entire network of the military camp—all without anyone's knowledge.

Strongholds work the same way in our civilian lives. Viewing pornography is a common way to invite evil into our lives, giving the demonic a stronghold.

Temptation: This is an attempt to cause, lead, or trap someone into sin (Matt. 4:1-11).

Unresolved Sin: This is a sin that only you know about and are unwilling to confess to someone you trust (Jas. 5:16, Eph. 5:12-17).

We have learned God's design for sex, marriage and the family. We also have discussed the spiritual aspects of marriage, along with God's definition of sexual sin. Let's now take our first look at the "sex spiral" itself.

CHAPTER 3

TRIGGER #1: AWARENESS

"QUIT STARING! YOU'RE DOING SO good! It's almost been a whole month!" This kind of conversation used to go on in my mind as I stood in line at the grocery store staring at the magazines in the checkout stand—you know, *Cosmo, GQ,* and, of course, *Sports Illustrated: Swimsuit Edition.*

Unfortunately, a month was about the longest I could ever go without looking at porn. It seemed to be my breaking point. I'd be minding my own business—"living the dream"—and then *BAM!* something would happen. A smile from a pretty waitress, a random thought out of nowhere, the smell of a fragrance, a song on the radio, or any kind of pressure at work could start my head spinning with sexual thoughts.

Porn made me feel good. It was how I dealt with life. It actually changed my mood and was a lot easier to hide than alcohol or drugs. Ultimately, porn became my subconscious friend—the only one I thought I needed. "She" was always there for me. When I had a good day, I could celebrate with "her." When I had a bad day, "she" would comfort me. "She" never said no and was always willing to do whatever I imagined.

What I didn't realize, however, was that over time, "she" started to control me. There became a time in our relationship when I stopped choosing "her," and "she" chose me. "She" eventually became the one in charge, dictating when and how I would spend my time. "She" became a powerful force in my life. I had willingly participated for so long that a moral and spiritual transaction seemed to have taken place. Jesus said it this way in Luke 11:34-36: ***"Your eye is like a lamp that provides light*** *for your body. When your eye is healthy, your whole body is filled with light. But when it is unhealthy, your body is filled with darkness. Make sure that the light you think you have is not actually darkness. If you are filled with light, with no dark corners, then your whole life will be radiant, as though a floodlight were filling you with light."*

This change in my life was so subtle. I didn't realize it until major consequences started to happen to my relationships, career, and health. Why didn't I stop looking at pornography when I first sensed there was a problem? In other words, why didn't I break off this relationship with "her"? Well, I thought I could fix it on my own. I thought I could just quit.

THE REALITY OF LIFE SETS IN

In Proverbs 27:19 (NIV) we read, *"As water reflects the face, so one's life reflects the heart."*[33] I had no idea the kind of person that I truly was. I had become the "fruit" of pornography itself. My life exhibited a reflection of the anger and abuse that I had willingly viewed as entertainment for two decades. I knew something was wrong with me, but I had no idea the character of my heart and the deception of my own mind.

Even if I had wanted to tell someone about my struggle, who would listen? I was so wrapped up in myself that I had only one friend. Truth be told, I really didn't want any other friends. I remember turning down opportunities to go to the movies or dinner with a small group of people for the sole purpose of staying at home with "her." Not only did I not have any friends, but I also didn't have a relationship with God. *But* if you had asked me if I was a Christian, I would have said, "Yes, of course." After all, I went to Catholic school, was an altar boy, prayed, took communion, went to confession, etc. How could I *not* be a Christian?[34] Just look at all the stuff I did growing up. However, Jesus says in Matthew 7:21-23:

---

[33] *The Holy Bible: The New International Version.* Grand Rapids: Zondervan, 2011.
[34] Please know that I'm not condemning the Catholic faith or our Catholic friends. This problem fell directly on me.

Trigger #1: Awareness

Not everyone who calls out to me, "Lord! Lord!" will enter the Kingdom of Heaven. Only those who actually do the will of my Father in heaven will enter. On judgment day many will say to me, "Lord! Lord! We prophesied in your name and cast out demons in your name and performed many miracles in your name." But I will reply, "I never knew you. Get away from me, you who break God's laws."

This is one of the scariest verses in scripture. I *thought* that I was a Christian, but I *thought* very wrong. Notice the wording—*"Only those who actually do the will of my Father."* What is the will of our Heavenly Father when it comes to sexuality? The apostle Paul tells us in 1 Thessalonians 4:3-5, *"God's will is for you to be holy, so stay away from all sexual sin. Then each of you will control his own body and live in holiness and honor—not in lustful passion like the pagans who do not know God and his ways."*

Wow, how crystal clear is that? I certainly was not in God's will. In fact, I was the pagan that Paul is talking about in this verse. I was kidding myself. No, wait, that's not strong enough. I *chose* to believe in a lie that said, "Yes, I'm a Christian, *but* I can still keep this porn thing for myself."

I believe it's entirely possible that the pandemic of pornography within the Church is due to people who *think* they are Christians, but are not. This is possibly the biggest fatal, eternal assumption of our generation. Once again, we need to look at the words of Jesus in Matthew 7:15-20:

Beware of false prophets who come disguised as harmless sheep but are really vicious wolves. You can identify them by their fruit, that is, by the way they act. Can you pick grapes from thornbushes, or figs from thistles? A good tree produces good fruit, and a bad tree produces bad fruit. A good tree can't produce bad fruit, and a bad tree can't produce good fruit. So every tree that does not produce good fruit is chopped down and thrown into the fire. Yes, just as you can identify a tree by its fruit, so you can identify people by their actions.

Sexual sin is *the* battle of our generation. We don't just have churches blatantly rejecting the authority of the Bible in this area, but rather entire denominations are losing their mind over it. False prophets, pastors, priests, and ministers teach half-truths. Their intention is to deliberately turn people away from the one true God and toward themselves. They leave out truth that seems to be inconvenient. Make no doubt about it—their motives are evil. We have plenty of false prophets—each with their own microphone for misguided and unfounded theology. They preach a message that is anti-Christ. They call evil *good* and good *evil* (Isa. 5:20). These people have the appearance of godliness but deny His power (2 Tim. 3:1-5).

Are you sitting under a false teacher? How do you know? Ask your pastor, priest or minister two questions:
1. Is the Bible the inspired, infallible, and inerrant Word of God? If he answers no, you have a problem.
2. What *is* marriage? If he gives you his opinion instead of quoting Genesis 2:24, then it's time to find a new, Bible-based church home.

AWARENESS

The first trigger in *The Sex Spiral* is *Awareness*. Awareness is *not* temptation, and it's *not* a sin. Awareness is simply taking notice. It's being consciously aware that you are overly-sensitive and susceptible to lust. It's at this moment that you are vulnerable and "aware" of your temporary state of weakness. Once you become consciously aware that you have a problem with lust, you must make a decision. This very moment is paramount because if you don't proactively choose to make a godly decision, then you will passively make an ungodly one. We read in Genesis 4:7, **You will be accepted if you do what is right. But if you refuse to do what is right, then watch out! Sin is crouching at the door, eager to control you. But you must subdue it and be its master."**

Being aware of the severity of your lust is a huge part of the discovery process. As you engage in this journey toward sexual sobriety, you'll notice just how chronic your problem is. For example, it took more than a year for me to *not look* in the rearview mirror when I passed a female jogger alongside the road. I literally had trained and conditioned my body to do so. The good news is that *The Sex Spiral* will allow you to start breaking those habits and creating new, godly disciplines as you become more aware of your thoughts, motives, and feelings.

OPTION 1: FLEE!

Think of awareness as the warning light on the dashboard of your car. It's telling you that there is a potential problem. In other words, it's "go-time" for you to become very aware of your surroundings. When triggered, ask yourself these questions:

- What exactly are you doing?
- Why are you doing it?
- What are you looking at?
- What are you feeling?
- How are you feeling?
- What are you thinking?
- What are you planning to do?
- What's your motivation and agenda?

If you have the desire to engage in what your trigger is offering, *flee* the situation immediately! Using my grocery store example—I would find another cashier to check out my groceries. If that was not an option, I could simply exit the line and walk around the store for a few minutes. If that didn't work, I could leave the store and come back later.

The reason that you must flee is because you haven't learned the self-control to stay. You literally become drunk with lust. King Solomon writes in Proverbs 7:21-23, *"So she seduced him with her pretty speech and enticed him with her flattery. He followed her at once, like an ox going to the slaughter. He was like a stag caught in a trap, awaiting the arrow that would pierce its heart. He was like a bird flying into a snare, little knowing it would cost him his life."*

We learn how to flee from the story of Joseph in Genesis 39:6b-13:

> *Joseph was a very handsome and well-built young man, and Potiphar's wife soon began to look at him lustfully. "Come and sleep with me," she demanded. But Joseph refused. "Look," he told her, "my master trusts me with everything in his entire household. No one here has more authority than I do. He has held back nothing from me except you, because you are his wife. How could I do such a wicked thing? It would be a great sin against God." She kept putting pressure on Joseph day after day, but he refused to sleep with her, and he kept out of her way as much as possible. One day, however, no one else was around when he went in to do his work. She came and grabbed him by his cloak, demanding, "Come on, sleep with me!" Joseph tore himself away, but he left his cloak in her hand as he ran from the house.*

I'm hedging my bets that most men would not turn down an opportunity to sleep with a powerful and beautiful woman. However, Joseph did. It certainly is possible for Christian men, and God shows us this as an example. Joseph *ran*! He didn't think. He didn't ask questions or quote Scripture. He *ran*! This is why fleeing your trigger is the fastest way to remove yourself from a situation you don't want to be involved in. As you continue to read Joseph's story, you'll find

Trigger #1: Awareness

out that even bad things can still happen with right decisions. But let's take a step back and learn from a major mistake on Joseph's part before the drama unfolded.

JOSEPH'S MISTAKE

Is there a way all of this drama could have been avoided? I believe so. Joseph's mistake was that he didn't talk to his boss, Potiphar. He didn't tell him that his wife was flirting with him. Awkward, I know, but Joseph is basically in a no-win situation either way. I get that. But was Joseph aware of her flirtatious behavior? Of course. Was he vulnerable to actually saying yes to her advances? You bet. Did Joseph think that her sexual nagging would stop? Possibly, but the reality is that her *looking* at Joseph moved to her *seducing* Joseph.[35] Sexual sin always escalates when not confronted. *Always.* In this instance, flirting turned to violence because misplaced passion often does.

So let's learn from Joseph's mistake. We must be willing to communicate the uncomfortable in order to prevent worse things from happening. Is it possible that Joseph could have avoided being accused of rape by Potiphar's wife and then thrown into prison if he would have talked to Potiphar man to man? Is it possible that Potiphar's wife has done something like this before?

REAL WORLD EXAMPLE #1

About five years into my journey toward sexual sobriety, my wife, Amy, and I were visiting some friends over the weekend. One night we were watching TV, and our friend was flipping through the channels. He landed on a show where two people were having sex. I was expecting him to change it immediately. He and his wife started to laugh, and their teenage daughter gasped, "Oh my gosh!" After maybe five to seven seconds (which seemed like an hour), I literally jumped off the couch and walked briskly to my room for the night, saying

---

35 Weiss, Dr. Doug. *Clean: A Proven Plan for Men Committed to Sexual Integrity.* Nashville: Thomas Nelson, 2013.

nothing to anyone. I must admit that I was a little anxious about what the breakfast conversation was going to be like, but I didn't care. Regardless, I fled. God had prepared me by making the willful and conscious decision to read His Word and spend quiet, devoted time with Him almost every morning for the past five years. Because of that time with the Lord, I was able to take immediate action in what I thought was a safe place. I was able to honor Him and my wife by fleeing.

REAL WORLD EXAMPLE #2

Ten years into my purity journey, I was asked to meet a pastor friend for lunch. I'd heard of the place he recommended but had never been. When I walked through the door, there were several young women standing by the hostess booth who were practically naked. I started to stammer, trying to explain that I was supposed to meet someone for lunch. After a second to grasp the fact that I was looking at nearly-naked women standing directly in front of me, I turned my head into the seating area, looking for my friend. Everywhere I looked, there seemed to be another nearly-naked waitress! I then looked back at the women at the hostess counter, who were now looking at me with scowls on their faces. I immediately turned around and fled, saying nothing more to the women.

I called my friend from the parking lot and asked, "Is this some kind of sick joke?"

He replied, "What are you talking about?"

I said, "I was just in the restaurant with all the girls."

"What?" He said, "I'm sitting down having an appetizer right now. Where exactly are you?"

I said, "I'm standing in the parking lot looking at the restaurant sign that reads _____."

The phone went silent, and then I heard a roar of laughter. "OOHH, NOOO! Not _____! I'm at _____!"

He whispered, "Did you actually go in there?"

"Yes!" I replied. "I had no idea. I'll be over in a second to choke you!"

Trigger #1: Awareness

So yes, there were two restaurants that just happened to have a very similar name in the same exact shopping plaza. Go figure. However, before I went over to the right restaurant, I called my wife, Amy, and told her what happened. The phone went silent again. In one of the most serious tones I've ever heard, she asked, "Are you okay?"

Right then, I felt the weight of my past plague me. Please understand, Amy doesn't know the "old" Dustin (Eph. 4:22-24). Sure, she sees bits and pieces that come out from time to time, but she doesn't know that guy. Her question and tone of voice came from a love that I've never experienced. It's only by God's grace that I was able to say, "Yes, babe, I'm fine, but I wanted to tell you exactly what happened."

My point in sharing these fleeing stories is to show you that freedom really is possible. This is not wishful thinking, nor do we need to touch the hem of Jesus' robe (Lk. 8:43-48). Freedom really can start today by applying this one biblical principle alone (Prov. 5:8, 2:16-22, 6:20-29, 7:1-27; 1 Cor. 6:18, 10:14; 2 Tim. 2:22). So yes, you can do this too. The reality is that you never know when something like this will take place, but you can bank on the fact that it will happen when you least expect it.

OPTION #2: CONFESSION

The apostle John writes in 1 John 1:9, **"But if we confess our sins to him, he is faithful and just to forgive us our sins and to cleanse us from all wickedness."** Confession changes everything. Think of this verse as the vertical portion (stipes) of the cross. Here we see that God is faithful when we are not. He not only forgives us, but He also doesn't hold our sin against us (Ps. 103:12). He actually purges us from evil each time we confess.

I can't tell you how many times I've confessed my sin to God in the midst of my "addiction." I would tell God, "Okay, Lord, I'm not going to do *that* again." Then the next day would come, and I would say, "Um, okay, Lord, I know that I told You that I would never do *that* again, but I did. Please forgive me." The next day turned into next month, which

66 THE SEX SPIRAL

then turned into a year, which then turned into two decades. Did God forgive me each time? Yes. He is the One who is faithful; I was not. So why wasn't I changing? Jesus' half-brother answered that question in James 5:16 (NIV): ***"Therefore confess your sins to each other and pray for each other so that you may be healed. The prayer of a righteous person is powerful and effective."***[36]

This verse is like the horizontal portion (patibulum) of the cross. Just as God forgives us vertically in 1 John 1:9, the verse in James holds the key to unlock the prison door by reaching out horizontally. Notice that James doesn't tell us to confess our sins to God. It's like he already knows we do that. When we learn how to confess a secret sin to a trusted, Christ-centered friend, the secret loses its power (Eph. 5:12-14).

Now some of you may be thinking, "Wait a second. Are you telling me that I must confess my porn and masturbation habit to someone else—like face-to-face?" Nope, I'm not saying it; God is. Look at the rest of the verse, *"so that you may be healed."* Confession is where your healing begins! Confession allows us to come out of hiding.

Back to my grocery store scenario—there I am, standing in line, waiting to pay for my groceries, and staring at the *Cosmo* magazine. I'm triggered, and I need to confess what I want to do next. So what do I do? I phone a friend (yes, just like the cheesy game show). I would pay for my groceries, get to my car, and call a friend. Now here's where the power of God through confession comes in. My friend may or may not answer my call. I may get voicemail. But the truth of God's Word through confession is so powerful that all I have to do is quickly tell my story in the voicemail, and the healing process will begin. Your friend's only job at that point is to call or text back, telling you how proud he is of you and that he loves you. It's very important that these phone calls don't turn into counseling or therapy sessions. If these phone calls turn into a list of things that should and should not be done, then the phone calls will cease because the friend is not safe. The trusted friend is to be exactly that—a friend, not a counselor and

---

36 *The Holy Bible: The New International Version*. Grand Rapids: Zondervan, 2011.

not a therapist (even if he is one.) There is a time for counseling, but it's not here.

Secondly, the type of confession that we're discussing here is the confession of the awareness trigger. It's not of the sin because we have not committed the sin yet. The goal of confession is to confess what you are thinking about doing, not what have you have already done. Your trusted, Christ-centered friend is not acting as a priest to where he absolves you of your sins, but rather a Brother who is walking your purity journey with you.

The psalmist writes about confession in Psalm 32:3-5.

When I refused to confess my sin, my body wasted away, and I groaned all day long. Day and night your hand of discipline was heavy on me. My strength evaporated like water in the summer heat. Finally, I confessed all my sins to you and stopped trying to hide my guilt. I said to myself, "I will confess my rebellion to the Lord.*" And you forgave me! All my guilt is gone.*

OPTION #3: PRAYER

Jesus tells us in Matthew 26:41, **"Keep watch and pray, so that you will not give in to temptation. For the spirit is willing, but the body is weak!"** The word *watch* in the Greek is used twenty-two other times in the New Testament. It implies "staying awake, being ready, and alert." It's translated "to have the alertness of a guard at night." A guard at night must have a different skillset than a guard during the day. He must rely on his other senses instead of just sight. He must be "hyper-alert" to keep him from being attacked. This is the type of prayer Jesus was referring to.

It's taken me forty-five years to learn how to pray. I used to tell God what to do during my quiet time for years. It's only when we discussed

James 1:5 during group one day that I realized that I had completely missed it all these years.

"If you need wisdom, ask our generous God, and he will give it to you. He will not rebuke you for asking" (Jas. 1:5). God will always give us *wisdom* when we ask. My problem with prayer was that I wasn't asking for wisdom; I was telling God how to do His job. Needless to say, that never worked out so well. I was telling Him how He could make my life easier, rather than simply praying, "God, will You please give me wisdom in how to handle this situation?"

Now you may be thinking, *But I* have *prayed, and I have asked for wisdom—for years, even decades, but it's like God refuses to answer.* If that is the case, let's turn to more Scripture to find out why (emphasis mine).

- Isaiah 59:1-2—**"Listen! The Lord's arm is not too weak to save you, nor is his ear too deaf to hear you call. It's your sins that have cut you off from God. <u>Because of your sins, he has turned away and will not listen anymore.</u>"**
- Proverbs 28:9—**"God detests the prayers of a person <u>who ignores the law.</u>"**
- 1 Peter 3:7—**"In the same way, you husbands must give honor to your wives. Treat your wife with understanding as you live together. She may be weaker than you are, but she is your equal partner in God's gift of new life. Treat her as you should <u>so your prayers will not be hindered.</u>"**

The other item that goes with prayer is memorized Scripture. Do you know the Lord's prayer? (Matt. 6:9-13). If so, pray this out loud when triggered. There is power in speaking God's Word *out loud*. After all, God spoke the universe into existence from nothing. The Old Testament prophets performed miracle after miracle with that same power. Jesus used this power to heal the blind and raise the dead. We have this same power! It carries authority from Christ Himself through the Holy Spirit.

Trigger #1: Awareness

At the end of the day you have a choice. You can either pray for someone or you can prey on them.[37] Praying for someone that you find attractive prevents you from preying on them and taking something from them that's not yours. It's hard to lust after someone when you are praying for them. I like to pray something like this: Father, there is a very attractive woman over there, and I want to lift her up to You. I praise You and thank You for her beauty. She is beautiful because You are, indeed, the Creator of all beauty. She is a reflection of Who You are. You created her in Your own image—of course she's beautiful! But, Father, there is a part of me who wants to look and lust. There is a part of me who wants to fantasize, but, Lord, I choose not to. I know that with You all things are possible. I know that Your grace is sufficient, therefore, I want to pray for this person and not prey on them. I pray for her soul, Lord God. I pray that she knows You and the salvation You offer. I pray for a godly man in her life to treat her as You treat her. I pray for her family, her home, and her health, Lord God. It's in Jesus' name I pray. Amen.

It is amazing what a sixty-second prayer like this will do in your life. You don't have to pray it word for word; I would encourage you to write your own and pray it aloud. Lastly, if all this seems overwhelming, I would encourage you to pray and repeat three short, yet life-changing words from the apostle John in Revelation 22:20b: ***"Come, Lord Jesus!"***

I DON'T KNOW IF I CAN DO THIS

What happens if you choose not to flee, confess, or pray when triggered? The next layer down the spiral is *unhealthy thoughts*. Essentially, it's shame. It's the unhealthy thoughts we tell ourselves as we go

---

37 Peter Bartolini, "Important Things About Men," (camp book for kids, 2007).

through this spiral. It's the voice that always tells us what a loser we are and how we'll never be anything.

When we refuse to exit a trigger, the winds of the spiral pick up speed and thrust us down further into the tornado where the winds become more powerful. This downward progression is inevitable because the lure of lust is inescapable, unavoidable, and irresistible when you choose to do nothing. Choosing to do nothing is, indeed, a very real choice we make. You are, in fact, allowing lust to choose you. The more your awareness intensifies *without* fleeing, confession, or prayer, the more your mind is consumed with lust.

Ultimately, the reason we don't want to flee, confess, or pray is because of our pride. The apostle Paul writes in 1 Corinthians 10:12-13: **"If you think you are standing strong, be careful not to fall. The temptations in your life are no different from what others experience. And God is faithful. He will not allow the temptation to be more than you can stand. When you are tempted, He will show you a way out so that you can endure."**

Notice three things about this verse. First, Paul is telling us that you can't do this alone. Secondly, those thoughts and fantasies that you're having are the same thoughts and fantasies experienced by *many other people as well*. Basically, God is telling you to quit believing the lie that you are the only one who thinks this stuff up.

Thirdly, notice the word *endure*. This means that God wants you to "go through the temptation," not around it. He wants you to *experience* the trigger and then make a *godly* decision by fleeing, confessing, and praying because this builds spiritual muscle as you learn to draw your strength from Him. If we continue to work within our own discipline, strength, and wisdom, we'll crumble every time because we don't have the *supernatural* strength to say no.

The apostle Peter writes in 2 Peter 2:9, **"So you see, the Lord knows how to rescue godly people from their trials . . ."** Think about the last time you were aware of your lust. How did God give you a way out? In this verse, we see that He does. Most of us, however, can't see

Trigger #1: Awareness

God giving us a way out because our mind immediately starts to think about the pleasure of lust rather than fleeing from it. If we choose not to flee, confess, or pray at this point, what happens? We move down the spiral another layer into shame—trigger #2.

CHAPTER 4

TRIGGER #2: SHAME

UNDERSTANDING THE TRIGGER OF *SHAME* is critical to understanding *The Sex Spiral* in its entirety. What we tell ourselves about ourselves really does matter. Most of us don't realize that we continue to make poor decisions on the most important events in our lives because of previous relationships. Our unhealthy thought life directly contributes to the weight of our shame. This could stem from a traumatic event that happened during childhood up to the present. Trauma is an experience that produces psychological pain. The most common form of trauma is through emotional abuse from the intentional words of critical parents or the lack of words from an absent parent.

Am I suggesting that bondage to pornography comes only from some sort of traumatic experience as a child? No, of course not. However, viewing pornography as a child certainly qualifies as a traumatic event. It's emotionally traumatic because most of us remember our first pornographic image to this very day. Secondly, we may have "flashbacks" and anger issues as an adult and not understand the root cause. Ultimately, we choose pornography because it provides pleasure. It's a temporary escape from the real world. If we didn't receive some type of pleasure from the behavior, we wouldn't engage—regardless of what we say to ourselves or others.

I've had many men say something like this over the years: "I used to gamble, drink, and do drugs, and I was able to quit all of those—some of them even 'cold-turkey'—so why is this porn thing different?" The answer is found in 1 Corinthians 6:18-20. The apostle Paul writes,

> *Run from sexual sin! <u>No other sin so clearly affects the body as this one does. For sexual immorality is a sin against your own body.</u> Don't you realize that your body is the temple of the Holy Spirit, who lives in you and was given to you by God? You do not belong to yourself, for God bought you with a high price. So you must honor God with your body* (emphasis mine).

Paul is saying that sexual sin is unique because every other sin is committed *outside* the body. In other words, gambling, drinking, and drugs certainly affect us emotionally and physiologically, but they do not affect the body spiritually like sexual sin. We are made in the image of God. Our bodies consist of our physical body, our spirit, and the Holy Spirit. This means that we are sexual *and* spiritual beings. Therefore, no other sin has the potential for bondage like sexual sin because we are attaching ourselves (the temple of God) to something that is profane.

Paul asks this question in 1 Corinthians 3:16, **Do you not know that you are God's temple and that God's Spirit dwells in you?"**[38] When we sin sexually, a spiritual transaction takes place. We are not just sinning against our physical body, but we are also sinning against our spirit and God's Spirit as well. Spiritual ties with the person or the object we are engaging with are also created and now must be broken. Yes, indeed, no other sin carries this kind of power. No other sin is more shameful. It's different, unique, and demonic for all the reasons we discussed in Chapter Two.

SHAME

Shame is the disgraceful feeling that exists from sin, failure, public exposure, and/or dishonor. It's a painful emotion that oozes humiliation and disgrace. Humiliation is something that causes emotional pain and guilt. It's usually something that very few people know about. Dr. Patrick Carnes, the founder of the term "sex addiction," discovered four belief statements that were consistent with his work in dealing with "sex addicts":

---

38 *The Holy Bible: English Standard Version.* Wheaton: Standard Bible Society, 2016.

Trigger #2: Shame

- I am basically a bad and unworthy person.
- No one will love me as I am.
- My needs are never going to be met if I depend on others.
- Sex is my most important need.[39]

As a redeemed "porn and sex addict," I don't ever remember consciously telling myself any of these four things. From a spiritual perspective, these belief statements are lies. Let's go over these lies individually so that you can become aware of them in your own life.

1) I am basically a bad and unworthy person.

If you would have suggested this to me, I'm pretty sure I would have been deeply offended and told you to go get wet. "I'm a pretty good guy, not a bad one. Sure, I'm not perfect, but who is? We all have our own flaws, right?"

The problem with my answer, however, is that my behavior told a very different story. Although I was blind to it at the time, my actions were not that of a person who was a "pretty good guy" or worthy to be trusted at any level. My behavior proved, without a shadow of a doubt, that I was indeed an unworthy person looking out for only myself, striving to be noticed. I was always yearning for my boss to tell me that I did a good job or seeking to impress a woman on the first date. Essentially, I handed over my worthiness and self-identity to other people. When I didn't live up to their expectations, it crushed me and then catapulted me into the sex spiral all over again.

2) No one will love me as I am.

When I didn't live up to someone else's expectations, this meant that I had to change something about myself. For example, I turned

---

[39] Carnes, Dr. Patrick. *Out of the Shadows: Understanding Sexual Addiction.* Center City: Hazelden Publishing, 1983.

into a chameleon—especially when dating. I was trying so hard for a woman to like me that I remember getting on a dating website and scheduling three dates in one day. I was binge dating (not only dumb, but very expensive). I ended up liking whatever my date liked because previous experience had taught me that I must change who I am. If I didn't, I would remain alone and unloved. The problem with my thinking is that I was putting on a front. I was wearing an invisible, fake mask to cover my real identity. The very thing I was trying to accomplish was working against itself because the love I was trying to receive was going to the mask I was wearing. The love never reached the real me.[40]

3) My needs are never going to be met if I depend on others.

This lie is one of the biggest reasons pornography is attractive in the beginning. It's the illusion of being in control and having needs met quickly. Pornography teaches that real sex and intimacy are too much work and that relationships are too difficult. This is why I can't depend on others. I'm not satisfied by what I'm receiving from them. Ultimately, porn teaches that God's design for sexuality is not worth the effort because we've grown so accustomed to the instant gratification of sex with ourselves that we wonder why we should even bother pursuing real relationships. Therefore, we continue to believe more lies—that life is just simpler this way and that it's a lot less drama.

4) Sex is my most important need.

This subconscious lie is one we will risk everything for to get our "fix." It's the reason we risk our jobs by viewing porn at work or on company devices. It's the reason we risk our marriage and our children's future by continuing the web of lies that surrounds our porn use. It's

---

[40] Thrall, Bill, Bruce McNicol, and John Lynch. *TrueFaced: Trust God and Others with Who You Really Are*. Colorado Springs: NavPress, 2004.

Trigger #2: Shame

the reason we risk our health and the health of our spouse by having unprotected sex.

If sex were not our most important need, why on earth would we risk so much for so little? As we'll soon discuss, pornography changes the very structure of our brains over time. This means that our decision-making is also greatly impacted. We honestly believe the lie that we'll never get caught. That's how powerful the sin of lust truly is. This reality is shocking. Ultimately, we spend time with the people and things that we love. It's really that simple. When you're in bondage to pornography, you will make time to spend with it and risk everything for a fantasy that will never come true. Even *if* your fantasy did come true, then what?

We must understand that these four beliefs are lies straight from hell. Believe it or not, there are demonic forces that surround you who want nothing less than to ruin your witness for Christ and/or take your physical life.

The apostle Peter gives a stark warning in 1 Peter 5:8: **"Stay alert! Watch out for your great enemy, the devil. He prowls around like a roaring lion, looking for someone to devour."** The word *devour* in this passage literally means to "gulp down." Have you ever seen a lion stalk and attack her prey? She is patient and strategic, and at just the right time—which is one of her prey's weakest moments—she attacks quickly and swiftly. Before you know what hit you, your job is gone; your marriage is in turmoil; and your relationships are devastated.

I received a dose of reality when my second "marriage" was over. It was more like a manic mirage as it lasted only five months. I married one of the women with whom I was committing adultery. This, by the way, is a sure sign of how sexual sin makes us stupid. One day as we were going through the actual divorce proceedings, she and a half dozen people that I didn't know stormed into the house and took most of the furniture. The only things left were a chair and a TV that sat on the floor. I remember sitting alone in what *seemed* to be a really big house. There was literally nothing in it. I then had this vision of Satan standing there laughing at me—as well he should. I believed him. I just stared back at him and couldn't believe that I had chased this lie of lust for two decades.

YOUR REAL IDENTITY

To overcome these lies, we must replace them with the truth of Scripture. We must constantly wash our mind with what is really true about us—regardless of how we feel. We must learn a new habit of filling our mind with Scripture to find freedom from pornography. The apostle Paul writes in Romans 12:1-2:

And so, dear brothers and sisters, I plead with you to give your bodies to God because of all he has done for you. Let them be a living and holy sacrifice—the kind he will find acceptable. This is truly the way to worship him. Don't copy the behavior and customs of this world, <u>but let God transform you into a new person by changing the way you think.</u> Then you will learn to know God's will for you, which is good and pleasing and perfect (emphasis mine).

Our behavior is followed by how we think. Our mind is where this battle begins. For example, if we choose happy thoughts, then our behavior will follow by smiling and laughing. If we think angry thoughts, then the opposite is true. We'll frown and be rude to people. The same is true with sexual thoughts. If we are preoccupied with sex, we'll *eventually* act out sexually. That's why the words from the apostle Paul are prophetic in Romans 8:5, **"Those who are dominated by the sinful nature think about sinful things, but those who are controlled by the Holy Spirit think about things that please the Spirit."** Paul encourages us in Philippians 4:8b, **"Fix your thoughts on what is true, and honorable, and right, and pure, and lovely, and admirable. Think about things that are excellent and worthy of praise."** If we don't allow the Holy Spirit to control our mind, then our flesh most certainly will.

From a physiological perspective, our brain is "plastic."[41] This means that although your porn use may have caused real physiological damage, God, in His grace, allows the brain to heal itself. The solution to healing your brain seems too good to be true. We simply need to change our habit of viewing porn and instead read the Bible from cover to cover, over and over.[42] The apostle Paul says it this way in Ephesians 4:22-24, ***"Throw off your old sinful nature and your former way of life, which is corrupted by lust and deception. Instead, let the Spirit renew your thoughts and attitudes. Put on your new nature, created to be like God—truly righteous and holy."***

This is where we learn what God says about us and where our true identity comes from. It comes from Him! It is often said that when you read God's Word, you're listening to His voice. So, regardless of what you've heard or what you've told yourself in the past, God says that you are:

- A new creature in Christ (2 Cor. 5:17);
- Chosen, holy, and blameless before God (Eph. 1:4);
- Sealed with the Holy Spirit (Eph. 1:13);
- Made complete in Christ (Col. 2:10);
- Justified and redeemed (Rom. 3:24).

YOUR SHAME STORY

When we first start reading what God says about us in the Bible, it's hard to believe, isn't it? First, we're offended to find out that we're no-good sinners and that there is nothing we could ever do to make things right—except for believing Jesus Christ as Lord and Savior (Acts 16:31, Rom. 10:9). Secondly, it's hard to believe that Jesus would love

---

41 Clinton, Timothy and Dr. Mark Laaser. *The Fight of Your Life: Manning Up to the Challenge of Sexual Integrity*. Shippensburg: Destiny Image Publishers, Inc., 2015.
42 Nair, Ken. "Discovering the Mind of a Woman." Workshop, Thomas Nelson, Nashville, 1995.

us so much that He casts all our sin and shame as far as the east is from the west (Ps. 103:12) by taking the punishment and death that we deserve. No matter how grateful we may be, many of us still grapple with this new kind of undeserved and unfathomable love. We tend to still struggle with a problem. The problem is called *shame*. We have lived the majority of our lives out of different shame stories, and although Christ cast it away, we still live with it. Your shame story is the combination of the harmful events in your life and how you choose to live your current life according to those unresolved past events. We may fluctuate back and forth between shame stories depending on whether we are at work or at home. We may even fluctuate between different people at work or home. Regardless, these shame stories are based on lies rather than on God's Truth.

1. **Strong Person:** If I'm the strong person in the relationship, then you're the weak person. And if you're the weak person, then you're the problem. Ultimately, if it weren't for you, I'd be just fine. In fact, you're the reason I choose to view porn and act out sexually.

2. **Weak Person:** Since I'm the weak person in the relationship, I really do believe that everything that happens is my fault.

3. **Wounded Person:** I've been hurt so many times, I expect it. No, it's much more than that—I *deserve* to be treated this way. I don't know how to be treated otherwise. When people do treat me with dignity, I run away believing that I don't deserve it.

4. **Godly Person:** My worthiness is based on how much I sin or don't sin. This is a *huge* theological problem absent of grace and based in works. It's one of the biggest reasons that Bible-believing, fundamental Christians keep their lust and pornography a secret for so long.[43]

Ultimately, when you combine the four false belief statements to your personal shame story above, you will continually make critical

---

[43] Steven Stack, Ira Wasserman, and Roger Kern. "Adult Social Bonds." *Social Science Quarterly*, 85 (2004): 75-88.

Trigger #2: Shame

life decisions based out of your shame. Your shame story will drive your compulsive behavior, and your lust will end up replacing God.

Your shame story is the reason that you can get whisked away into the winds of the sex spiral. Apart from physiological or medical reasons, there's really nothing else but shame that drives your bondage to pornography. You can actually go through all twelve triggers in a matter of minutes, months, or years. I personally found myself going through this spiral a half dozen or more times per day for years.

Shame is the reason why pornography is so powerful. The shame of being exposed as a liar and pervert is often stronger than the guilt of living in perversion. Until the pain of life begins to outweigh the shame, we rarely come forward in full disclosure. We'll hide and lie until we're caught or don't have a choice because of circumstances beyond our control. Even then, it'll take years for the whole truth to come out because of our shame. I believe the lie that I can't do anything about it because I haven't—nor will I ever—lived up to God's purity standards.

Just because this trigger is where shame begins doesn't mean that's where it also ends. Jesus conquered shame to give you a new, shame-free identity. Jesus did not come *primarily* to stop us from sinning. He came primarily to give us a new identity so that we, by our own choice, could and would stop sinning. Now, make no doubt about it, God wants us to stop sinning (Jer. 26:13, Dan. 4:27, Jn. 5:14, 1 Cor. 15:34). Jesus gave His life to break the power of sin within us, but how is it done? Is it done by keeping the Ten Commandments? Nope, the law was to reveal the rebellion in our hearts (Rom. 7:7-12). Ultimately, our lust problem is a heart problem, and our heart problem is a God problem. It's been this way from the beginning of humanity, but by God's grace we read:

"I will give you a new heart, and I will put a new spirit in you. I will take out your stony, stubborn heart and give you a tender, responsive heart" (Ezek. 36:26).

"I will give them a heart to know that I am the LORD, and they shall be my people and I will be their God, for they shall return to me with their whole heart" (Jer. 24:7, ESV).[44]

JESUS & SEXUAL SIN

I'm personally heartbroken and, at the same time, infuriated at the dichotomy between how Jesus spoke to sexual sinners and how His Church does today. In John 4, we see an amazing conversation between Jesus and a Samaritan woman. I'm struck at the effort Jesus made to even get to Samaria to speak to this woman. I'm also amazed at the length of the conversation itself. Overall, Jesus really didn't have long conversations with people other than His disciples. There are exceptions, of course, but my point is that Jesus went well out of His way to minister to a pagan, sexual sinner. (This is like the Church going out of its way to minister to a convicted Muslim sexual offender.)

Talk about a woman filled with shame. Jesus knows that she has been married five times and is living with someone who is not her husband. This woman has had six lovers. She has gone from man to man, searching for love and intimacy, but finding only pain. She didn't know that the Lover she had been looking for her entire life was standing right in front of her! Jesus was the seventh man in her life,[45] but He was offering her a new kind of love—to be the Lover of her soul. At the end of the conversation, Jesus doesn't give her a three-point sermon telling her to stop sinning. He doesn't give her a list of the things that she *should* be doing and another list of the things she *should not* be doing. Oh, no. He actually tells her that He is indeed *the* Messiah—the Husband she's been searching for! In doing so, He told her all the things she needed to hear so that she could and would stop sinning.

---

44 *The Holy Bible: English Standard Version.* Wheaton: Standard Bible Society, 2016.
45 West, Christopher. *Your Body Tells God's Story: An Intro to St. John Paul's II, "Theology of the Body,"* Audio CD. https://shop.corproject.com/cds/cd-your-body-tells-god-s-story.html.

Trigger #2: Shame

In John 8, we read about a woman caught in the very act of adultery. Imagine this scene:

They are caught in the very act, and pastors break into the house to stop the crime. The pastors then drag this woman (not the man) through the church on the way to *kill her.* She's in shock, crying, pleading, screaming, all with no clothes on or *maybe* a sheet wrapped around her. The pastors are more than willing to carry out God's law on this subject—to pummel stones at her until she's dead. They would be right in doing so because that's the law (Lev. 20:10). But on their way to joyfully execute this woman, they just happen to run into Jesus and ask His opinion. Jesus says in John 8:7 (ESV), **"Let him who is without sin among you be the first to throw a stone at her."**[46]

Can you imagine the silence? It must have been strangely silent. This woman now has a second chance at life because Jesus is the only One who could actually throw that first stone. This is called "amazing grace"—a grace that was unfathomable in Jesus' day and a grace that we seem to extend only to acceptable sins in our churches today (like gluttony and gossip). Now, let's not miss where Jesus' grace leads to. In John 8:10-11 (ESV), Jesus says, **"'Woman, where are they? Has no one condemned you?' She said, 'No one, Lord.' And Jesus said, 'Neither do I condemn you; go, and from now on sin no more.'"**[47]

What this woman didn't know is that this very same Jesus was on His way to Calvary to die for her shame and adultery. This woman was specifically instructed to "go and sin no more." How does she do that? How do you do it? We can only sin no more because of a heart transplant conducted by Jesus Christ Himself when He willfully and purposefully gave His life as a substitute for ours.

Jesus did not come *primarily* to stop us from sinning, He came primarily to give us a new identity *so that* we could and would stop sinning by our own volition. Once we have this spiritual heart transplant, everything changes. EVERYTHING! It's only then that we can get our

---

46 *The Holy Bible: English Standard Version.* Wheaton: Standard Bible Society, 2016.
47 Ibid.

I'M A CHRISTIAN AND I WATCH PORN

Everyone who sins is breaking God's law, for all sin is contrary to the law of God. And you know that Jesus came to take away our sins, and there is no sin in him. Anyone who continues to live in him will not sin. But anyone who keeps on sinning does not know him or understand who he is.

Dear children, don't let anyone deceive you about this: When people do what is right, it shows that they are righteous, even as Christ is righteous.

But when people keep on sinning, it shows that they belong to the devil, who has been sinning since the beginning. But the Son of God came to destroy the works of the devil.

Those who have been born into God's family do not make a practice of sinning, because God's life is in them. So they can't keep on sinning, because they are children of God (1 Jn. 3:4-9).

If you have been struggling with pornography and call yourself a Christian, the above words of the apostle John are terrifying. I would encourage you to read them again and again. The apostle Paul also writes in the last part of Philippians 2:12 (ESV), **"Work out your own salvation with fear and trembling."**[48]

The Scriptures are crystal clear. *Do not be deceived.* Just because we call ourselves Christians, that doesn't mean that we really are. Time, trials, and temptations are the great purifier as to whether we are who we say we are. This is where we feel the tension of who we once were versus who we are now. Our hearts are redeemed, but the rest of our bodies are not. We can be a Christian and in bondage to pornography at the same time, but God's Word tells us that we can't stay there for long (Rom. 6). Christians possess the power of God through the Holy

---

48 Ibid.

Spirit, and this power is the same power that raised Jesus Christ from the dead. If the Holy Spirit can do that, then He can certainly free you from the bondage of pornography.

THE SEVEN PLACES

In 2003, I bought a CD from a Christian rock band called Seven Places.[49] One of the tracks on this CD was a snippet of a sermon by Pastor Jon Courson. On this track, he explained the seven places that Jesus Christ bled from on the way to Calvary. To this day, that track makes me weep. The picture was crystal clear—even though I had spent more than twenty years of my life as a sexual sinner, I still could be forgiven and free in Christ.

The book of Isaiah was written 500 to 700 years before Christ was even born. In Isaiah 52:14, he writes about Jesus, *"But many were amazed when they saw him. His face was so disfigured he seemed hardly human, and from his appearance, one would scarcely know he was a man."*

Did you know that Jesus Christ bled from seven places on the way to Calvary to forgive your (sexual) sin? Why did Jesus have to bleed? According to Hebrews 9:22, *"In fact, according to the law of Moses, nearly everything was purified with blood. For without the shedding of blood, there is no forgiveness."*

The First Place: Jesus' Head

(Matt. 27:29, Mk. 15:17, Jn. 19:2)

Roman soldiers took their time to twist together and create a *crown of thorns*. Placing the crown of thorns on Jesus' head was meant to not only bring tremendous pain, but also to humiliate Jesus as earthly kings wear crowns of gold and jewels. Now keep in mind that Roman soldiers were perfecters of pain, so they forced the crown onto Jesus' head and beat it into His skull with a wooden walking stick called a

---

49 Seven Places, *Lonely for the Last Time*. BEC Recordings, 2003.

"reed or staff." They continued mocking Him by giving the staff to Jesus as a "scepter." A scepter is a symbol of supreme power. The mocking then continued as they bowed before Him.

I want you to start looking into the rearview mirror of your life. Think about your thought life. Think about your fantasies—sexual and nonsexual. I want you to ponder all the things that you couldn't face up to in your past. Jesus Christ allowed the thorns to pierce His head in order to free you from those thoughts and fantasies. His blood cleanses you of your thought life, and, because His blood flowed from His head, you are forgiven for those sins.

The Second Place: Jesus' Back

(John 19:1)

The second place Jesus Christ bled from was His back. After the Roman soldiers got tired of mocking Jesus with the crown and scepter, they tied Him to a pole. They continued to beat Him with a *flagellum*[50]—a short whip made of leather ropes connected to a handle. The leather ropes were knotted with a number of small pieces of metal, usually zinc and iron, attached at various intervals. The flagellum was designed to quickly remove the skin of its victims. The soldiers beat (also known as flogging or scourging) Jesus beyond human recognition.

The prophet Isaiah predicted this account in Isaiah 50:6: ***"I offered my back to those who beat me and my cheeks to those who pulled out my beard. I did not hide my face from mockery and spitting."*** I want you to now think of how you have turned your own back on God by running away and doing your own thing. Jesus' blood flowed from His back, and you are now forgiven.

---

[50] Davis, C. Truman , MD., M.S. "A Physician's View of the Crucifixion of Jesus Christ." CBN.com. http://www1.cbn.com/medical-view-of-the-crucifixion-of-jesus-christ (accessed January 2014).

Trigger #2: Shame

The Third and Fourth Places: Jesus' Hands

(Matt. 27:35, Lk. 23:33, Mk. 15:24, Jn. 19:18)

After Jesus was forced to carry His own cross to what is called "The Place of the Skull" or Golgotha, Roman soldiers took metal spikes and nailed His hands to the cross.

I want you to think about how many times you have used your own hands to view pornography and masturbate. How many clicks of the mouse? How many swipes with your tablet or phone? I want you to think about the people that you touched that you should have never touched—whether it was for sexual pleasure or out of anger. Those actions and behaviors are the reasons that Jesus' hands were nailed to the cross. His blood flowed for you, and you are now forgiven.

The Fifth and Sixth Places: Jesus' Feet

(Matt. 27:35, Lk. 23:33, Mk. 15:24, Jn. 19:18)

The Romans soldiers took another metal spike and pinned Jesus' feet to the cross. I want you to think about how many times you have walked where you should have never walked. How many times have you run into the arms of your adulteress? Once again, Jesus' blood flowed for you, and you are forgiven.

The Seventh Place: Jesus' Side

(Jn. 19:33)

One of the soldiers took his spear and thrust it into the side of Jesus, piercing His heart. Both blood and water flowed from His side. Blood and water are signs of a dead man. It's what you get during an autopsy. It's also a symbol of the New Covenant—a new life in Christ.

Finally, I want you to think about the anger, resentment, and unforgiveness that you hold inside towards God and others. Yes, Jesus bled from His side, too, which means you are forgiven.

The prophet Isaiah predicted all of this in Isaiah 53:5: ***"But he was pierced for our rebellion, crushed for our sins. He was beaten so we could be whole. He was whipped so we could be healed."***

IT IS FINISHED

Earlier we discussed that sin is a debt that must be paid. Here, we've learned that Jesus Christ paid that debt. The wrath that God had toward you and your sexual sin has been paid in full. Jesus Christ bled from seven places, physically died, and chose to raise Himself from the dead—to conquer death once and for all. God is not mad at you for your sexual sin and doesn't punish you for it. That punishment—that retaliation (Matt. 5:38)—of God seeking justice for the injustice (sexual sin) that you committed toward Him has been paid in full by Jesus Himself. When Jesus said, "It is finished," He meant that He alone absorbed the rightful punishment and wrath of your sin (Jn. 19:30). He was made sin so that we could have a relationship with His Father (2 Cor. 5:21). Therefore, there is no more shame and guilt for those who have accepted Jesus Christ as Lord and Savior (Rom. 8:1).[51]

Does this mean that there are no consequences for acting out with sexual sin today and tomorrow? Of course not, there will be severe *discipline* involved, but not punishment. Both punishment and discipline involve pain, but discipline is to educate, reform, and protect us from future pain.[52] It's to grow us. These consequences that we experience deal with God's discipline, as a loving father disciplines His own child (Prov. 3:11-12, 13:1, 15:10, 22:15).

The apostle John wrote the most familiar verse in the Bible, John 3:16 (ESV): ***"For God so loved the world, that he gave his only Son, that***

---

[51] https://dustindaniels.org/2017/03/01/difference-discipline-punishment.
[52] Murray, Karis Kimmel. *Grace Based Discipline: How To Be At Your Best When Your Kids Are At Their Worst*. Phoenix: Family Matters Press, 2017.

*whoever believes in him should not perish but have eternal life."*⁵³ This is an excellent time to ask the Lord into your life or recommit your life to Him. Maybe you thought you were a Christian but now realize that your behavior condemns you. Regardless, there is no special prayer or formula to ask the Lord Jesus into your life. Simply confess your sins to Him. Tell Him that you have rebelled and turned away from these sins and that you are right now calling on His name—Jesus Christ—to save you.

The apostle Paul also writes in 2 Corinthians 5:17 (ESV), *"Therefore, if anyone is in Christ, he is a new creation. The old has passed away; behold, the new has come."*⁵⁴ Since the new has come, this means we need a new plan to deal with old temptations. Let's move into Trigger #3 and learn what temptations really are.

---

53 *The Holy Bible: English Standard Version.* Wheaton: Standard Bible Society, 2016.
54 Ibid.

CHAPTER 5

TRIGGER #3: TEST / TEMPTATION

"WHAT'S THE DIFFERENCE BETWEEN A trigger and a temptation?" Aaron asked in one of my classes. "I feel like I'm just tempted and have never gone through the triggers of awareness and shame. It's like I'm tempted, and I automatically sin, and that's it."

"Do you look at porn *every time* you're tempted?" I asked.

Aaron smirked and replied, "Well, no . . . not *every* time. If I did, I'd never leave the house!"

I continued, "So if you don't look at porn every time you're tempted, then is your sin really automatic?"

Aaron hesitated and said in a low, sheepish voice, "Nooo."

I then pressed on, "If it's not automatic, then it sounds to me like you have a choice, correct?"

"Wow, I guess so," Aaron responded.

TRIGGERS VS. TEMPTATIONS

Triggers and Temptations are similar, but let's go over the specific differences. It's important that we understand these differences, so we know exactly where we are in the sex spiral. Once we know where we are, then we can start making godly decisions to exit the spiral itself.

Trigger: A person, thing, or event that makes me aware of being vulnerable to potentially questionable behavior. A trigger could be anything—an attractive person, a picture on a magazine, a song on the radio, a certain aroma, a thought that jumped in your mind, a good day at work, a bad day at work, a traffic jam, etc. It's important to know that a trigger is not a temptation or a sin, but it can certainly lead to that when not addressed immediately. Triggers explain the location as to where you are *right now* in the "sex spiral" and are the precursor to temptation.

Temptation: An attempt to cause, lead, or trap someone to sin (Matt. 4:1-11). Temptation is a choice fueled by desire. This choice reveals the nature of a person. It's where we experience tension. This tension between the trigger and the temptation is what most of us run from. Unfortunately, this is a mistake. God doesn't want us to go around the test or temptation. He wants us to go straight through it by experiencing the full weight of it.

PUTTING IT ALL TOGETHER

In my previous example of waiting in line at the grocery store, my trigger was the *Cosmo* magazine. I became *aware* of it while standing in line. I simply noticed it. I didn't do anything wrong. But due to my propensity for lust, it now caused tension. Once again, noticing someone or something is not sin. It just feels that way because of the way I've responded in the past. However, temptation quickly enters *when I make the choice* to keep looking at the magazine. When I continue to look (or take a second or third look), I begin to separate the person from her sexuality. I divorce her body from her personhood. *This* is the moment that lust enters, and I commit sexual sin. When I allow my mind to become preoccupied with sex, that preoccupation propels me into looking at pornography later in the day if I choose not to flee, confess or pray.

Trigger #3: Test / Temptation

TRIGGER → TENSION → TEMPTATION

DECISION

DESIRE

Am I going to flee, confess, or pray?

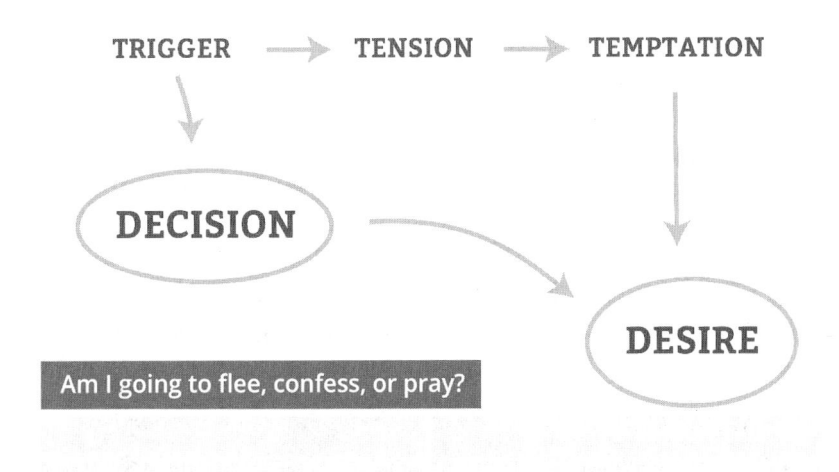

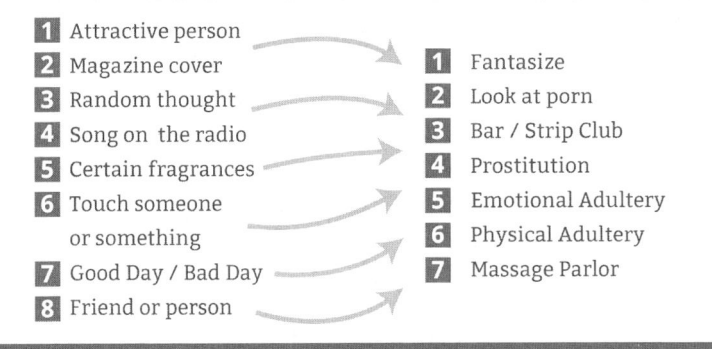

1. Attractive person
2. Magazine cover
3. Random thought
4. Song on the radio
5. Certain fragrances
6. Touch someone or something
7. Good Day / Bad Day
8. Friend or person

1. Fantasize
2. Look at porn
3. Bar / Strip Club
4. Prostitution
5. Emotional Adultery
6. Physical Adultery
7. Massage Parlor

A trigger is the precursor to the temptation. The temptation is our desire to fulfill it.

Back to my class, Jack blurted out, "I wish Satan would just stop tempting me all the time!"

Jack's response is all too common. We give Satan way too much credit for our temptations. First and foremost, Satan is not simply the evil version of Jesus. Satan is a created being by God. Jesus is God—the second person of the Trinity. Therefore, Satan is not omnipresent, so he can't be everywhere at one time like God (Job 1:6-7, Matt. 4:3). I'm pretty sure Satan is busy running a demonic empire rather than individually tempting working slugs like you and me to look at porn. That's not to say he doesn't have demons that do so, because he does (Rev. 12:4, 9; Jude 6). However, my point is this—most of our temptations actually come from *ourselves,* not Satan nor demons.

Jesus' half-brother writes in James 1:14-15, **"Temptation comes from our own desires, which entice us and drag us away. These desires give birth to sinful actions. And when sin is allowed to grow, it gives birth to death."** Do you see the mini-spiral in this verse? Submitting to temptation leads to sinful behavior, and sinful behavior with no resolve gives birth to emotional, spiritual, and physical death.

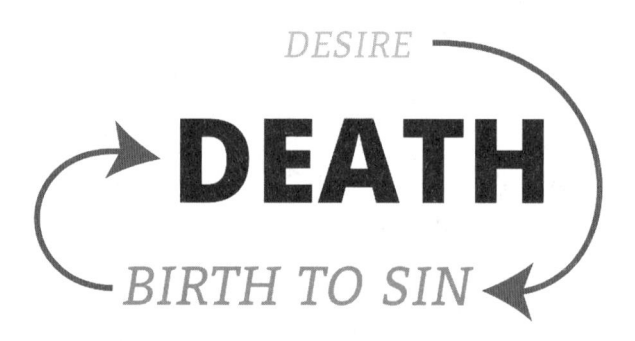

DESIRE → **DEATH** → *BIRTH TO SIN*

From the back of the class, Patrick asked, "How do we get to the point like you did where we're not tempted anymore?"

I started laughing and asked, "Who told you that I'm not tempted?"

Patrick tried to refrain from smiling.

I continued, "Would it surprise you that I'm tempted every single day? In fact, many times per day—just like you. If I were a gambling man, I would place a bet that I'm probably tempted more than you because I'm teaching God's design for sex, marriage, and the family. The demonic would rejoice if I were to fall. Here's the thing—sexual temptation is universal to every single person, but victory over temptation is not. In fact, testing and temptation are critical keys that unlock the door to personal holiness. How else would you know that you're growing into the character of Christ? Besides, the more mature we become in Christ, the more attuned we become—not just to lust but to sin in general."

Jesus said in Matthew 18:7b, *"Temptations are inevitable, but what sorrow awaits the person who does the tempting."* James 1:3-4 also says, *"For you know that when your faith is tested, your endurance has a chance to grow. So let it grow, for when your endurance is fully developed, you will be perfect and complete, needing nothing."* It's through these tests that we build spiritual muscle. Testing and temptations are where the proverbial "rubber meets the road." It's where our theology meets reality. If married, you most likely have told your spouse "I'm sorry" a gazillion times. You've promised her that you will indeed "change," but how does this change take place?

The prophet Isaiah writes profound words in Isaiah 28:10: *"He tells us everything over and over—one line at a time, one line at a time, a little here, and a little there!"* He's telling us that moral change takes place over time by reading the Bible cover to cover, over and over![55] It's learning His commands and then applying His commands on top of previous commands. Being tested sexually is God's way of changing you and your moral character. In fact, it's the only way to change (Jn. 14:6). I would encourage you to embrace the test and go on the offensive (flee, confess, or pray) instead of retreating and acting defensively. Too many times, we pray for God to take the temptation away. *He won't.* Look at what Jesus told the apostle Paul after he begged for relief:

> *Three different times I begged the Lord to take it away. Each time he said, "My grace is all you need. My power works best in weakness." So now I am glad to boast about my weaknesses, so that the power of Christ can work through me. That's why I take pleasure in my weaknesses, and in the insults, hardships, persecutions, and troubles that I suffer for Christ. For when I am weak, then I am strong* (2 Cor. 12:8-10).

---

55 Ibid.

JESUS AND TEMPTATION

Did you know that Jesus was tempted? *"Then Jesus was led by the Spirit into the wilderness to be tempted there by the devil"* (Matt. 4:1). The Greek word for "tempted" in this verse is *peirasmós* (per-ahz-mos). It is a neutral word which means that it can be used as a testing for good *or* a temptation for evil.[56] From God's viewpoint, this is a test as He never tempts anyone. Jesus' half-brother writes in James 1:13, *"And remember, when you are being tempted, do not say, 'God is tempting me.' God is never tempted to do wrong, and he never tempts anyone else."* From Satan's perspective, however, it's a temptation. Luke states in Luke 4:13, *"When the devil had finished tempting Jesus, he left him until the next opportunity came."*

In other words, God provides an opportunity to prove that you are growing in sexual integrity by offering a test; but from the devil's standpoint, it's a temptation to trap or trick you into sin. Satan intends this situation for evil, while God intends it for good (Gen. 50:20). The issue with being tested or tempted is that you can't really see the difference until you experience the outcome. If I pass, then it's a *test* that proves that I'm learning how to be a person of sexual integrity. If I fail, then it's a *temptation* in which I was enticed by my own lust and chose to sin.[57]

It's important to note that Jesus was always in conflict with Satan and people, yet never sinned (2 Cor. 5:21, Jn. 8:46, 1 Pt. 2:22, Heb. 4:15). Not only was Jesus tempted in *every* way, but He was tempted to the absolute highest limit of temptation. Think of temptation levels on a scale from one to ten.

---

[56] MacArthur, John. "The Temptation of Christ." GracetoYou.org. https://www.gty.org/library/sermons-library/90-84/the-temptation-of-christ (accessed April 23, 1995).
[57] Ibid.

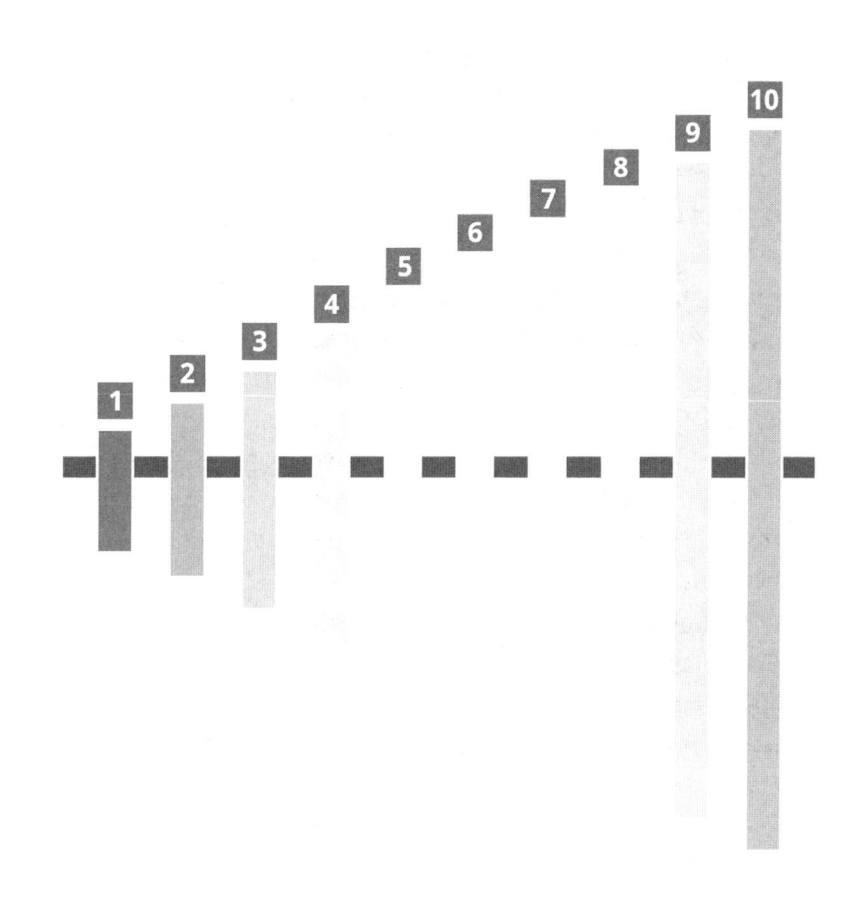

Jesus never gave into temptation. Not once. As the Son of Man, Jesus did what Adam could not do. Jesus says in Matthew 5:17, *"Don't misunderstand why I have come. I did not come to abolish the law of Moses or the writings of the prophets. No, I came to accomplish their purpose."*

In other words, Jesus fulfilled every law. As each test/temptation presented itself, it had to become more powerful and seductive than the previous one. This continued throughout Jesus' life until all temptations reached level ten.[58] We see this most apparent in the Garden of Gethsemane.

Matthew 26:39 states, *"He went on a little farther and bowed with his face to the ground, praying, 'My Father! If it is possible, let this cup of suffering be taken away from me. Yet I want your will to be done, not mine.'"* As the Son of Man (a human being), Jesus was praying that His Father would remove the suffering that was about to take place. His temptation was to quit. It was to step out of the Father's will and not have to experience the pain of His destiny.

"Then Jesus left them a second time and prayed, 'My Father! If this cup cannot be taken away unless I drink it, your will be done'" **(Matt. 26:42).** This second prayer from Jesus is not a different version of the first one. Jesus is not begging His Father to make His life easier. He realizes that His Father said no to His prayer. In response, Jesus prays for His Father's will to be done once again. Do you see the increase in tension within each temptation? This is how we know that Jesus' grace is sufficient when we cry out to Him.

According to Hebrews 4:14-16, *"So then, since we have a great High Priest who has entered heaven, Jesus the Son of God, let us hold firmly to what we believe. This High Priest of ours understands our weaknesses, <u>for he faced all of the same testings we do, yet he did not sin.</u> So let us come boldly to the throne of our gracious God. There we will receive his mercy, and we will find grace to help us when we need it most"* (emphasis mine). We may give into temptation at a three or four on the scale and stay at that level for years and even decades without ever passing that particular threshold. As we mature over time, we will embrace God's beautiful plan for purity in our lives *through* testing and temptations (1 Cor. 13:11). We cannot go around these events in our lives. It is God's will that we experience the full weight as we walk through them.

In fact, God has predestined that you go *through* these tests, temptations, and trials. In Romans 8:29 (ESV), the apostle Paul writes, *"For*

---

58 Ibid.

Trigger #3: Test / Temptation

those whom he foreknew he also predestined to be conformed to the image of his Son . . . "[59] Paul writes again in Ephesians 1:4-5 (ESV), *"Even as he chose us in him before the foundation of the world, that we should be holy and blameless before him. In love he predestined us for adoption to himself as sons through Jesus Christ, according to the purpose of his will."*[60]

For us to grow in sexual integrity, we must feel the full weight of each test. Just as Jesus clung to His Father in the Garden of Gethsemane, we are to cling to Christ as we go through our tests as well. As an athlete gets stronger, more weights must slowly be applied to his workout routine. The same principle applies to us spiritually. To build spiritual muscle, we must get our eyes off the sin and onto our Savior by embracing these tests and temptations rather than running from them.

STRONGHOLDS

The apostle Paul in 2 Corinthians 10:3-5 reminds us, *"We are human, but we don't wage war as humans do. We use God's mighty weapons, not worldly weapons, to knock down the strongholds of human reasoning and to destroy false arguments. We destroy every proud obstacle that keeps people from knowing God. We capture their rebellious thoughts and teach them to obey Christ."*

What mighty weapons is Paul referring to in this passage? *Prayer and the Bible.* Are you using these weapons on a daily basis? Have you destroyed *every obstacle* that keeps you from knowing God?

Doing nothing is an invitation for all sorts of evil to come into our lives. Oh, how the demons love our passivity. When it comes to strongholds, this is where we have to deal with the demonic head-on. First Peter 5:8 reads, *"Stay alert! Watch out for your great enemy, the devil. He prowls around like a roaring lion, looking for someone to devour."*

Viewing pornography is the easiest way to invite a stronghold into your life. With every click of the mouse, every image, every desire, and

---

59 *The Holy Bible: English Standard Version.* Wheaton: Standard Bible Society, 2016.
60 Ibid.

every act of masturbation, the chains get heavier. Proverbs 5:22 warns, **"An evil man is held captive by his own sins; they are ropes that catch and hold him."**

Viewing pornography is like leaving the front door to your home wide open so the demons can physically walk in and crash on your couch. Make no doubt about it—pornography is evil, and where evil is, the demonic live. Strongholds don't appear overnight. They are built over time. For example, I didn't just wake up one day and decide to commit adultery on my first wife. It took over twenty years. This stronghold started in childhood with my eyes. As an adolescent, I looked at women who were not mine. As a young man, I then allowed sexual fantasies to take over my mind. Then, as an adult, I allowed the pleasure of lust to push my moral boundaries around, which then led to more sinful actions. All of these decisions led to a lifestyle of sexual attachments and, finally, bondage.

Sexual temptation is simply a detour from God's best and highest plan for your life because it gives you the opportunity to enjoy the pleasure of lust. It's at this time that you choose to believe or not believe the lies we previously discussed:

- I am basically a bad and unworthy person;
- No one will love me as I am;
- My needs are never going to be met if I depend on others;
- Sex is my most important need.

Then you add in the shame story of yourself:

- I am a strong person;
- I am a weak person;
- I am a wounded person;
- I am a godly person.

We can *choose* not to believe these lies. Part of this purity journey is learning how to replace lies with God's truth. It's not easy, and it was never intended to be, but it is a choice. You can start changing today by the grace of God. After all, the apostle John writes in 1 John 4:4, *"... The Spirit who lives in you is greater than the spirit who lives in the world."* The apostle Paul also writes in Romans 8:31b-32, *"If God is for us, who can ever be against us? Since he did not spare even his own Son but gave him up for us all, won't he also give us everything else?"*

Of course, God will give us everything else! In fact, He's already given it to you. He's already destined that you live a porn-free life. You just may not realize it yet.

UNASHAMEDLY HONEST

The writer of Hebrews 11:24-25 states, *"It was by faith that Moses, when he grew up, refused to be called the son of Pharaoh's daughter. He chose to share the oppression of God's people instead of <u>enjoying the fleeting pleasures of sin</u>"* (emphasis mine).

Isn't it interesting how unashamedly honest God's Word actually is? The unknown writer of Hebrews states that sin is indeed pleasurable, *but* only for a short time. The pleasure of your lust is temporary, yet insatiable. Regardless, temptation now gives you the opportunity to enjoy the pleasure of sin. In other words, the temptation now creates an environment so that you can spend time with your adulteress. The temptation provides the right set of circumstances so that you can indulge in the pleasure of your lust.

Many of us don't want to admit what I just said. We don't want to admit that we're actually waiting to be tempted or that we long for an excuse to be tempted, and that's the reason we refuse to confess, flee, or pray. The longer I wait, the weaker I become because I'm consumed with the *pleasure* of sin. We also don't want to admit that the decision to not quickly confess, flee, or pray is, indeed, a decision to sin.

THE WORLD'S WISEST MAN

I find it fascinating that the world's wisest man—King Solomon—couldn't control his lust. Have you ever really thought about this? The world's wisest man lacked self-control. We read about it in 1 Kings 11:1-3:

> **Now King Solomon loved many foreign women. Besides Pharaoh's daughter, he married women from Moab, Ammon, Edom, Sidon, and from among the Hittites. The Lord had clearly instructed the people of Israel, "You must not marry them, because they will turn your hearts to their gods." <u>Yet Solomon insisted on loving them anyway.</u> He had 700 wives of royal birth and 300 concubines. And in fact, they did turn his heart away from the Lord** (emphasis mine).

A concubine is a woman who has a formal relationship with one man (her husband) but has less rights than a wife. A concubine's status with her husband was based on sexual pleasure. She was one step away from a prostitute, but the husband provided for her daily needs. She was ultimately a sexual slave that had family rights.

Why on earth did King Solomon have 700 sex slaves? One word—*disobedience*. King Solomon had the knowledge of God but refused to apply it to his own life. He could tell you what to do, but he couldn't do it himself. Does this sound familiar? I've heard many stories of men leading "purity groups" who didn't have sexual sobriety themselves. That's evil! Does that make *any* sense to you? Would you take financial advice from someone who is going through bankruptcy? Fitness advice from someone who is obese? Of course not. These people can't give you what they don't have.

Solomon's life exhibits firsthand the insatiability of lust. Just exactly how many women does it take to satisfy a man? God purposed only one (Gen. 2:24). It's been said that a man's wife is his personal standard for beauty, which is true. But for Solomon, he believed the lie that more is better, and had 1,000 wives. Let's think about this: Solomon had 1,000 women that were at his disposal. He could have sex with a different woman every day for two-and-a-half years before seeing the first woman again. Every sexual fantasy known to man had come true for King Solomon. In Ecclesiastes 2:10a, Solomon admits, *"Anything I wanted, I would take. I denied myself no pleasure."* Yet his disobedience brought great misery to his life. Why? Because Solomon couldn't control the temporary, physical pleasure that lust brings. He knew the truth, but he just refused to apply it. Solomon wrote Proverbs 5:23, which turned out to be prophetic, *"He will die for lack of self-control; he will be lost because of his great foolishness."*

THE PROCESS TO PURITY

The Sex Spiral presents a process to sexual sobriety and integrity. This process is critical to understand. You can live without looking at pornography for a time; but without truly dealing with your lust head on by learning the disciplines of fleeing, confessing, and praying, the spiral will swipe you off your feet and throw you headlong into the next trigger. If you make the effort to address this, you will be a very different person next year. Yes, this may sound extreme at first. It will be inconvenient. You will feel like a child at times, but God doesn't want you to stay here. He has so much to show you as you grow past this first phase. He wants you to experience what it's like to have a normal conversation with a beautiful woman by looking into her eyes and not at her body.

The process to purity includes a "hyper-awareness" to your sexual triggers and a hatred of passivity. In order for you be tempted, you actually have to give yourself permission to be tempted. When you give yourself permission to be tempted, you are giving yourself permission to disobey God and to dishonor others. Let's now turn the page to see what happens when we try to resist sin on our own.

CHAPTER 6

TRIGGER #4: RESISTANCE

WHAT DO YOU THINK THIS is? Take a close look...

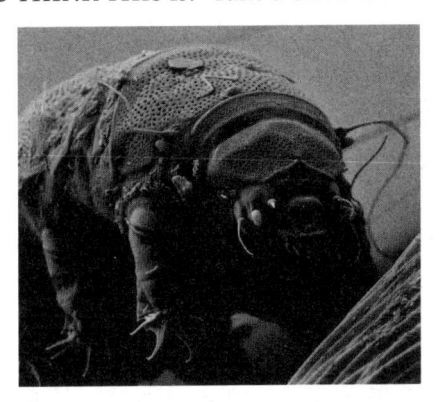

Let me introduce you to a *Tardigrade*. It's also known as a water bear or moss piglet. Tardigrades are microscopic, water-dwelling animals with eight legs.[61] Tardigrades can survive temperatures from as low as -459°F to as high as 303°F (that's 1,000 times more radiation than other animals). Tardigrades can also live almost a decade without water.

Even more impressive, in September 2007, Tardigrades were taken into orbit on the FOTON-M3 space mission and were exposed to space for ten days. After they were returned to earth, it was discovered that many of them not only survived, but also had laid eggs that hatched normally. Tardigrades are the only animals known to be able to survive the vacuum of space!

---

61 Ledford, Heidi. "Spacesuits Optional for 'Water Bears.'" Nature.com. http://www.nature.com/news/2008/080908/full/news.2008.1087.html (accessed September 8, 2008).

WHY DO YOU CARE?

When it comes to resistance, lust is like a tardigrade. Over the years, you have more than likely tried to stop looking at pornography many times. Maybe you were able to quit other sinful behaviors like drinking, drugs, gambling, and overeating. But as you have found out, pornography is different, isn't it (1 Cor. 6:18)?

You want to stop, so you've researched online for the best books. You have prayed more, read the Bible more, visited Bible studies, joined church retreats, and even tried counseling. You've had some success of staying clean for a few weeks, months, or even a year or two; but for some odd reason, your enslavement to pornography just doesn't seem to go away. Why?

Pornography is like a tardigrade. No matter what you've tried to do to resolve your porn problem *on your own*, that dang tardigrade just keeps coming back into your life. An unresolved sin like lust can be quiet for a certain period of time. It can even appear dead at times. But because there wasn't any resolution (a true commitment or plan involving godly community), it wasn't even close to being dead. Just when you thought that you touched the hem of Jesus' robe (Matt. 9:21), and He miraculously healed you . . . *BAM!* you find yourself in the spiral once again.

We've learned that it is not the sin any longer but rather *the pleasure of that sin* that you're in bondage to. You may love Jesus; but if you're in this spiral, you simply love your pleasure more. How do you know? By your behavior. We spend time with the people and/or the things we love. Skipping your devotional time in the morning because you "don't have time" but taking the opportunity to look at porn at work or at night proves who you love more. I know that's a hard pill to swallow, but it's true. Examining your actual day-to-day behavior is critical to becoming free. The apostle Paul encourages us in 2 Corinthians 13:5, **"Examine yourselves to see if your faith is genuine. Test yourselves. Surely you know that Jesus Christ is among you; if not, you have failed the test of genuine faith."** The prophet Jeremiah also urges us in Lamentations 3:40, *"Instead, let us test and examine our ways. Let us turn back to the Lord."*

Confessing that you love porn more than Jesus is a monumental step in the right direction. Confessing that you simply don't want to read the Bible in the morning instead of lying to yourself about time management is epic. Once we really start getting honest with ourselves, then we realize just how depraved our hearts really are. The prophet Jeremiah writes these revealing words in Jeremiah 17:9-10, *"The human heart is the most deceitful of all things, and desperately wicked. Who really knows how bad it is? But I, the Lord, search all hearts and examine secret motives. I give all people their due rewards, according to what their actions deserve."*

RESISTING INCORRECTLY

This trigger of resistance is where many of us think the real battle is won or lost. We think the godlier I am, the better I'll be at resistance—but then you haven't met a tardigrade until now. We think that resistance is the *only* point of victory or defeat. We believe that our decision, based right here, will be controlled by our godliness. This is a lie; don't believe it. Don't over-spiritualize what needs to happen for you to start breaking free (fleeing, confessing, and praying).

When we hear the word *resistance*, we may think of the following Scriptures:

- Ephesians 6:11—*"Put on all of God's armor so that you will be able to stand firm against all strategies of the devil."*
- 1 Peter 5:8-9a—*"Stay alert! Watch out for your great enemy, the devil. He prowls around like a roaring lion, looking for someone to devour. Stand firm against him, and be strong in your faith."*

The problem in dealing with habitual sin like pornography and using verses like these for recovery is that we're not using the whole counsel of God. When the Lord speaks directly on the subject of sexual sin, He doesn't use the terminology of "standing firm." He specifically uses terms like *flee, run, stay away, don't associate, don't indulge*, etc.

- 1 Corinthians 6:18—***"Run** from sexual sin! No other sin so clearly affects the body as this one does. For sexual immorality is a sin against your own body."*
- 2 Timothy 2:22 (ESV)—***"So flee youthful passions** and pursue righteousness, faith, love, and peace, along with those who call on the Lord from a pure heart."*[62]
- Colossians 3:5—*"So **put to death** the sinful, earthly things lurking within you. **Have nothing to do** with sexual immorality, impurity, lust, and evil desires."*

This is why it's so critical to flee or confess your trigger. In the beginning of this purity journey, you do not have the self-control to withstand the temptation. That's why God uses words like *flee, run,* and *avoid*. Even if you "white-knuckle" your temptations by being victorious for a short period of time, what tends to happen when you finally do cave in? The pleasure of your sin is escalated. Why? *Extended resistance only intensifies the pleasure.* As I mentioned before, the longest I could resist viewing porn seemed to be only one month at a time. When I finally gave in, the pleasure was even more pleasurable than normal.

THE IRONY OF SIN

If resistance intensifies the pleasure of sin, resistance has now become an enemy to your purity. In other words, *resistance* (standing firm) is now working against you. Your definition of resistance is now in opposition to the very thing you're trying to achieve! Why? You have learned how to increase the pleasure of sin—the very thing you can't control.

---

62 *The Holy Bible: English Standard Version.* Wheaton: Standard Bible Society, 2016.

RESISTING BIBLICALLY

When you learn how to resist sin biblically, you're learning how to build spiritual muscle slowly over time. *Putting on the full armor of God* (Eph. 6:10-20) speaks to spending time with the Lord by reading, listening, and meditating on His Word during your devotional time. This is a scheduled time of preparation between you and the Lord. The practice of resistance is not only done while the test is happening, but also in the quietness and solitude of your devotional time. Let me suggest to you the idea of *tithing your time*.[63] Just like we give the first ten percent of our finances to God as an offering for His provisions (Mal. 3:10), we can learn to tithe the first ten percent of our day as well. For example, if you plan on working eight hours for the day, you would literally schedule (tithe) forty-eight minutes as your devotional time before you start your work day.

Once again, it's not just in the thick of the battle that we learn resistance, but also on our face every morning before the Lord. Now, please don't hear what I didn't say. Yes, you will need to resist the test/temptation as it happens. My encouragement to you is to not let that be the only time for resistance itself. The test *is* coming for you. You're not going to stop it, but you can learn how to correctly resist it.

OBEYING YOUR WORD

I prefer the concept of a "prayer retreat" rather than a "devotional time." It's a time of quietness, safety, and solitude with the Holy Spirit. It's a time of relationship building, spiritual education, and preparation for the day. God has given us a structure for learning and applying sexual purity principles in Psalm 119:9-16. He first asks the question, answers it in the same verse, and then lays out a structure to follow.

How can a young person stay pure? By obeying your word.
¹⁰ I have tried hard to find you—don't let me wander from

---

[63] My mentor, Mark R. Miller, taught me this prayer concept through his Truth at Work roundtable groups.

your commands. ⁱⁱ I have hidden your word in my heart, that I might not sin against you. ¹² I praise you, O Lord; teach me your decrees. ¹³ I have recited aloud all the regulations you have given us. ¹⁴ I have rejoiced in your laws as much as in riches. ¹⁵ I will study your commandments and reflect on your ways. ¹⁶ I will delight in your decrees and not forget your Word.

As we read this passage we notice six things:

1. Verse 11—To hide God's Word in our heart, we must spend time with Him to develop the relationship.
2. Verse 12—To come with an attitude of worship.
3. Verse 13—To read God's Word out loud.
4. Verse 14—To come with an attitude of thankfulness.
5. Verse 15—To think deeply and critically on God's Word, to mediate, ask questions, challenge, and journal.
6. Verse 16—To actually enjoy this time and not to rush through it.

Reading Psalm 119 for forty days in a row would be a huge jump start to sexual sobriety. Keep a journal nearby to write down the things the Lord shows you.

If I choose not to flee, confess, or pray at this point, then I'll start talking myself into committing the sin. It's called *rationalization,* and it's our next trigger down the sex spiral.

CHAPTER 7

TRIGGER #5: RATIONALIZATION

YOU WOULD THINK THAT AFTER twenty years of telling myself the same things over and over that I would figure out that what I've been doing was not working. Some people call it insanity, but God calls it death in Proverbs 14:12: *"There is a path before each person that seems right, but it ends in death."*

Rationalization is talking yourself into committing the sin. It's what we tell ourselves *before* the sin. Justification (Trigger #9), on the other hand, is the excuses we tell ourselves *after* the sin. We rationalize what we are getting ready to do and justify what we just did. Both rationalization and justification make no sense to the person listening because both triggers are, in fact, irrational. These excuses that we tell ourselves are beyond ludicrous because we tend to tie unrelated events together, yet they make complete sense to us at the time. When we rationalize sin, we tend to think about or describe our thoughts and behavior in a way that makes it seem more attractive than it really is. The irony, of course, is that there is no rational explanation for engaging in sin. What we are really saying is "I want to, and you can't tell me that I can't."

It's important to note here that we usually are rationalizing to ourselves. If we were to talk to a godly person about the actual conversation that takes place in our heads, they would talk some sense into us. We may or may not listen, but that's not the point. The point is that most of us usually don't have long, extended conversations with ourselves during this time of rationalization. It usually ends up being one excuse that takes less than a second to choose, and then we move right onto Trigger #6—Concealment. This trigger is that quick; it's within a snap of a finger, and our decision is made.

There are countless rationalizations when it comes to pornography and masturbation. To understand the rationalization, we must understand the lie and then replace the lie with God's truth.

Below is a list of rationalizations that I have used myself and continue to hear today. These rationalizations are in no particular order. Once you recognize your sin of rationalization, it is very important to call a trusted friend and confess so that you can exit the spiral.

1. **I've had a good day, so I'll celebrate.** This is a "catch-all" excuse. What exactly are you celebrating, and who are you celebrating with? The reality is that you are looking forward to spending time with your "friend," pornography.

2. **I've had a bad day, so porn will comfort me.** This is a half-lie. Pornography will comfort you only *momentarily*. From a physiological perspective, the dopamine and adrenaline will certainly alter your mood, but *only* temporarily. We must know that there is no long-term comfort or healing in isolation. To be truly comforted means to engage in a real, authentic, face-to-face conversation with a Christ-centered, trusted friend. I find it incredibly interesting that one of the most unusual punishments within the prison system is solitary confinement. Although you are not in a physical prison, you *choose* to make your home, office, room, or car into your own personal prison cell by willfully choosing to isolate yourself from society. Your phone, tablet, or computer has become a metaphor for the prison chains around your ankles.

3. **I'm sad, mad, or frustrated, so porn will make me feel better.** This is a half-lie and is similar to the above rationalization. Once again, the truth is that pornography will make you feel better only temporarily. Pornography seems to be the new drug of choice. After all, you don't have to stick a needle in your arm, nor do you have the smell of alcohol on your breath. However,

without the saving grace of Jesus Christ and a humble obedience toward a purity plan, we tend to go back for more of the new drug—just like an alcoholic going back for a drink or a drug addict taking another pill. *"As a dog returns to its vomit, so a fool repeats his foolishness"* (Prov. 26:11).

4. **I'm not hurting anyone.** Yes, you are! You are hurting yourself in three specific areas:

    a) You are hurting your relationship with God by watching abuse take place by people who are made in the image of God.

    b) You are hurting yourself by not engaging in true, authentic relationships and conversations.

    c) You are fueling the activities of adult cabarets, prostitution, and human trafficking.[64]

5. **No one is getting hurt.** Wrong. *Everyone* involved in pornography gets hurt. They can't *not* get hurt emotionally, spiritually, and physically. Have you ever watched an interview with an ex-porn star? The abuse that happens to them on and off the photography or video set is demonic.

6. **The people on the screen like it.** Who told you that? Most women on the screen have been abused as a child or have run away from home. The men on the screen are abusers themselves. The reason these "actors" participate in this type of abuse is for the money to survive.

7. **Porn stars get paid lots of money.**[65] I guess it depends on what your definition of "a lot" actually is. People starting in the porn industry make approximately $300 per scene. The more dehumanizing the sex act, the more money they make. Here's my question to you—so what? What difference does income make

---

64 Countryman-Roswurm, Karen, "Why Fighting Sex Trafficking Absolutely Includes Fighting Pornography." FighttheNewDrug.org. http://fightthenewdrug.org/fighting-sex-trafficking-absolutely-includes-fighting-pornography/ (accessed May 24, 2017).

65 Morris, Chris. "Porn's Dirtiest Secret: What Everyone Gets Paid." CNBC.com http://www.cnbc.com/2016/01/20/porns-dirtiest-secret-what-everyone-gets-paid.html (accessed June 10, 2016).

at all? The truth is that you would still watch pornography if they chose to do it for free. This is one of the reasons "amateur" porn is so popular. You don't care about them. You only care that these "actors" cater to your every sexual desire.

8. **No one will ever know.** This lie comes from straight from hell.

   a) You know.

   b) God knows.

   c) If you're married, your spouse knows. She may not know exactly what's wrong yet, but she will.

- Psalm 44:21—***"God would surely have known it, for he knows the secrets of every heart."***
- Luke 8:17—***"For all that is secret will eventually be brought into the open, and everything that is concealed will be brought to light and made known to all."***
- Proverbs 10:9—***"People with integrity walk safely, but those who follow crooked paths will be exposed."***
- Ephesians 5:11-12—***"Take no part in the worthless deeds of evil and darkness; instead, expose them. It is shameful even to talk about the things that ungodly people do in secret."***
- Ecclesiastes 12:14—***"God will judge us for everything we do, including every secret thing, whether good or bad."***
- Hebrews 4:13—***"Nothing in all creation is hidden from God. Everything is naked and exposed before his eyes, and he is the one to whom we are accountable."***

God is right now, at this moment, allowing you to repent before He exposes your secret sin. He seems to make a habit of humiliating people if they do not repent. For example, Matt came to my office after he lost his job. He was completely horrified and humiliated as he was giving a PowerPoint presentation in front of potential clients and co-workers when a pornographic video "all of a sudden" just started to play.

Trigger #5: Rationalization

Terry, on the other hand, was a pastor of a medium-sized church that was growing. His I.T. person saw that something was wrong with the network. After spending some time diagnosing the problem, the I.T. person, along with a few members of the church staff, decided to walk into the worship center—only to find Pastor Terry watching a pornographic video on the large worship screens.

There are hundreds of stories that could fill this space, but I share only those two examples to emphasize the importance of humbling yourself before God humiliates you. God loves you too much not to expose your sin. I have found eight stages of habitual sin to be true in our lives: ignorance, rebellion, wooing, breaking, humility, cooperation, intimacy, and evangelism. Which stage do you find yourself in today?

9. **Everybody does it.** Everybody? Really? Do the statistics show that one hundred percent of all men and women are looking at porn? No, of course not. God called you to be holy, which means that you are set apart from the rest of the world. You are different; and if you are hanging around friends who make you think "everyone is doing it," it's time to leave those friends. The apostle Paul writes in 1 Corinthians 15:33 (ESV), ***"Do not be deceived: 'Bad company ruins good morals.'"***[66]

10. **It's my life and I can do what I want.** This statement is actually true if you *have not* accepted Jesus Christ as your Lord and Savior. However, if you have, then Scripture is crystal clear about this statement in the following passages:

    - 1 Corinthians 6:20—***"For God bought you with a high price. So you must honor God with your body."***
    - Jeremiah 10:23—***"I know, Lord, that our lives are not our own. We are not able to plan our own course."***

---

66 *The Holy Bible: English Standard Version.* Wheaton: Standard Bible Society, 2016.

- 1 John 3:16—*"We know what real love is because Jesus gave up his life for us. So we also ought to give up our lives for our brothers and sisters."*

11. **Nobody can tell me what to do with my body.** God can and does. Your physical body is no longer yours. It's His. The apostle Paul writes in 1 Corinthians 6:19-20, **"Don't you realize that your body is the temple of the Holy Spirit, who lives in you and was given to you by God? You do not belong to yourself, for God bought you with a high price. So you must honor God with your body."**

12. **My spouse said no, and I have needs.** What you actually mean is that you have "rights." This is one of the many great evils that porn teaches—to demand sexual fulfillment now. As Christians, we are to give up those rights (Phil. 2:6-8). Regardless, your spouse also has needs. Do you know the reason she said no? Is she not feeling well? Does she need to talk to you at a deeper emotional and spiritual level before becoming intimate? As we have learned, sex is not *just* physical. We must learn how to have social intercourse before sexual intercourse. Is God also trying to teach you how to be more emotional and spiritual *through* sexuality? Men often miss this because we refuse to listen to our wives. The apostle Paul writes in Philippians 2:4, **"Don't look out only for your own interests, but take an interest in others, too."**

13. **I'm single, and I have sexual needs.** No, you are single, and you have sexual *desires*. Are you willing to learn how to deal with those desires God's way or your way? King Solomon writes in Song of Songs 2:7b, *"... not to awaken love until the time is right."*

14. **It's okay to masturbate if I think about my spouse.** What Scripture verse confirms this? I hear this rationalization from a lot of men who travel because of their job. Does this behavior fit inside the template of sexuality as defined in Genesis 2:24? We convince ourselves of this lie because we Christians have bought

Trigger #5: Rationalization

into the world's theology on sexuality. We think it's actually proper to fantasize about our spouse (rather than someone else) and then act out while isolated and alone. After all, we convince ourselves that we're not watching porn, going to the strip club, or hiring a prostitute, right?

No, no, no! Your spouse is a *person* made in the very image of God. She is not a sex toy for you to consume. Also, these fantasies about your spouse tend to be of a more radical nature. In other words, you would not normally treat your wife in person the way that you fantasize with her in your head. We must remember that *any* sexual activity outside the covenant of marriage between one biological man and one biological woman is called *sin*. This implies that both husband and wife are physically together experiencing each other in sexual union. (See Chapter One.)

15. **Once I'm married, I'll stop.** Single people are usually shocked to learn that marriage actually tends to escalate the use of pornography and masturbation. Pornography use escalates during the first several years of a new marriage because self-control was not learned as a single person. If you were able to break God's commandment when single, then you certainly have the capacity to break your marriage vows to your spouse. All it takes is a set of right circumstances.

For example, did you pressure your spouse to have sex before marriage? If you did not have the self-control to wait for marriage, what makes you think that you will have the self-control when another woman begins to flirt with you after a long day at work or while in a fight with your spouse or as you travel across the country?

If you are willing to break God's laws as a single person, you certainly have the capacity to break your marriage vows. At this point, you may be thinking, *Not me. I did the former but won't do the latter.* Well, unfortunately, that's what I said, too, but I failed miserably . . . twice. Marriage and children bring on a new set of stresses—stresses that are supposed to make you godly and build moral character. However, if you have a false belief that your spouse is now going to fulfill the role of being your real-life porn toy, you will be severely mistaken.

For example, when she says, "No, I'm tired" or "I have a headache," you must be prepared to not fall back into your old habit as a single person. Lust has taught you that you deserve what you want, when you want it, and how you want it. The stresses of marriage not only have the tendency to escalate porn use but also devastate more people when it's brought into the marriage. A lot of times, your sin stems from your retaliation for her saying no to you in the first place.

16. **It's unhealthy not to masturbate.**[67] This is a myth. Many of us falsely believe that we will somehow physically explode. That's simply not true. Did you know that masturbation can be associated with symptoms of depression and prostate abnormalities? Excessive masturbation while watching pornography can also cause porn-induced erectile dysfunction (PIED) along with many other medical problems. For example, do you find yourself irritated for no particular reason? Do you fight depression? Masturbation could be a major factor. The truth is that God has given us a natural way for the body to relieve itself. It's called "nocturnal emission." It's also known as a "wet dream." So, no, you will not explode. I'm living proof of that.

17. **It's totally normal to masturbate.** It's one thing to experiment as a teenager; it's another to continue the practice into a habit. The bigger question here is, "Why?" At the end of the day, whatever excuse you give yourself is a smokescreen for the temporary pleasure it provides.

---

[67] Gilkerson, Luke. "The Great Masturbation Hoax: Is Not Masturbating Unhealthy for You?" Covenanteyes.com. http://www.covenanteyes.com/2015/04/13/the-great-masturbation-hoax-is-not-masturbating-unhealthy-for-you/ (accessed July 22, 2016).

18. **This will clear my mind.** It actually does the very opposite. It will make you feel guilty, angry, and/or lethargic.
19. **I've already started to lust/fantasize; I might as well follow through.** Making a godly decision *at this moment* is where we learn to change. This is the tension—the spiritual weights that are needed to build spiritual muscle. Learning to take these exact thoughts captive (2 Cor. 10:5) and run to the foot of the cross is where the frontline of this battle is engaged! It's *right here* where you can make the decision to change. It's *right here* where you can learn godly self-control and experience a changed life in Christ.
20. **I don't watch the hardcore stuff.** What's your definition of "hardcore"? What's your definition of pornography? Regardless, it doesn't matter. Keep watching, and you'll get there soon enough.
21. **Just one more time, and then I'll stop.** Didn't you tell yourself that yesterday, last week, or last month? The bigger question is, *Why can't you stop?*
22. **I'll watch porn but won't masturbate.** Yes, you will. You're just delaying the pleasure with resistance. (See Chapter Four.)
23. **I'll masturbate but won't watch porn.** No, you're choosing to not watch *new* porn. You're simply thinking of old porn in the library of your mind.
24. **I have an overly-sensitive sex drive.** No, you have a sinful propensity to lust.
25. **It's not like I'm at the strip club; it's better than picking up a prostitute; I'm not having an affair at work.** A big part of rationalization is comparing yourself to people who are far worse than you. As Christians, we are to compare ourselves only to Jesus Christ.
26. **Fantasy novels, *Cosmopolitan* magazine, and the *Sports Illustrated Swimsuit Edition* aren't really porn.** What is your definition of porn? In Matthew 5:28, Jesus defines porn for us: *"But I say, anyone who even looks at a woman with lust has*

already committed adultery with her in his heart." The problem with this verse, of course, is that we refuse to believe it.

27. **It's safer than real sex.** It's impossible to get an STD if you are having sex only with your spouse (and there is no drug use involved). In fact, STDs could be completely removed from society in one generation if we abstained. The same is true with pregnancy. If you are having sex only with your spouse, then there is no need to worry about unwanted pregnancies with other women.

28. **I don't care if I get caught.** At this point, we are letting our behavior speak for us and hoping we get caught, so the real conversation can begin.

29. **God will forgive me.** Wrong. God has already forgiven you. Dieterich Bonhoeffer called this attitude "cheap grace"[68] because you expect forgiveness without repentance. We are mocking the very gift of Jesus' blood that freed us from this very sin by using the gift of grace against itself.

    - Romans 6:1-2—*"Well then, should we keep on sinning so that God can show us more and more of his wonderful grace? Of course not! Since we have died to sin, how can we continue to live in it?"*
    - Galatians 5:1—*"So Christ has truly set us free. Now make sure that you stay free, and don't get tied up again in slavery to the law."*
    - Galatians 5:13—*"For you have been called to live in freedom, my brothers and sisters. But don't use your freedom to satisfy your sinful nature. Instead, use your freedom to serve one another in love."*
    - 1 Peter 2:16 (ESV)—*"Live as people who are free, not using your freedom as a cover-up for evil, but living as servants of God."*[69]

---

[68] Bonhoeffer, Dieterich. *The Cost of Discipleship.* New York: MacMillian Publishers, 1959.
[69] *The Holy Bible: English Standard Version.* Wheaton: Standard Bible Society, 2016.

Trigger #5: Rationalization

30. **Things are so messed up in my life, I might as well continue.** This excuse is on the verge of hopelessness. We tend to think that things can't get any worse. Depression sets in, and so do suicidal thoughts. These thoughts are lies. Life can always get worse, and with pornography, it most definitely will. The opposite is also true. Things can also get better. The healing comes from taking your eyes off yourself and putting them onto your Savior Jesus Christ.
31. **We're just messing around. We're not going to go that far; I can stop at any time.** It is often said that your past behavior is the best predictor of future behavior. The reality is that you *know* your whole agenda. Your intention is not to stop, and you certainly don't have the self-control. If you did, you wouldn't have started in the first place.
32. **I'm a great husband, and I provide for my wife and kids, so I deserve some time to myself.** This excuse allows us to use our time for evil and not good. Ask your wife, children, boss, and pastor if looking at porn is an example of what great husbands do in their spare time.
33. **I'll start tomorrow; someday, I'll be a "good Christian."** There is no such thing as a "good or bad Christian." However, we can be *obedient or disobedient* Christians. You get to choose.

Once we choose our rationalization, we move immediately into Trigger #6—*Concealment,* in preparation for acting out in sin.

CHAPTER 8

TRIGGER #6: CONCEALMENT

I USED TO HAVE A routine when I arrived home from work. I would walk my dog, eat dinner, and watch TV. I would then carefully and methodically shut my window blinds and curtains to watch pornography for hours upon hours until late night or early morning. But here's the thing: I didn't just make sure the blinds were shut; I would physically walk outside and look through all the windows to make sure no one could see in. I wanted complete and total privacy because I didn't want anyone (and I mean *anyone*) knowing what I was about to do. Trigger #6 is Concealment. My appetite for lust *demands* that I now hide to conceal my behavior.

ADAM HID

Genesis 3:8-10 reads, **"When the cool evening breezes were blowing, the man and his wife heard the Lord God walking about in the garden. So they hid from the Lord God among the trees. Then the Lord God called to the man, 'Where are you?' He replied, 'I heard you walking in the garden, so I hid. I was afraid because I was naked."**

Genesis 3:10 is one of the saddest verses in all of Scripture. Adam *hid*. He was *afraid* of God. Before the Fall, Adam had *no reason* to fear anything. He had this incredibly special relationship with God as they walked together in the garden.

From the very beginning, God intended life to be about relationships. God wanted us to experience life with Him and with others through deep, personal relationships. From the very beginning of humanity, God has also given people the ability to make choices. God did not create humans as robots or golden retrievers. Humans are different from animals because of the morality that God breathed into us (Gen. 2:7). These moral choices have eternal consequences.

God made it crystal clear to Adam of the one thing he was not to do in Genesis 2:16-17: **"But the Lord God warned him, 'You may freely eat the fruit of every tree in the garden—<u>except</u> the tree of the knowledge of good and evil. If you eat its fruit, you are sure to die.'"** The Lord's words here are emphatic. God *commanded* Adam. It's the same style of writing when God gave Moses the Ten Commandments. God is saying, "You will die—you will *surely* die—both physically and spiritually. Death will happen if you choose to disobey this *one* command."

Do you think Adam had any questions after that conversation? Did Adam ask what death was? Did Adam debate God on whether He had the right to tell Adam what to do? Was Adam confused at any level? Nope. Adam, however, willfully and consciously rebelled against God. Ultimately, we are talking about *disobedience*.

Have you ever thought about how many other trees were in the Garden of Eden? Hundreds maybe, possibly thousands, perhaps even tens of thousands! Regardless, Adam made a conscious, sinful decision that affected all of humanity. Take notice that Adam and Eve *hid* themselves from God after they experienced evil. Can you imagine *that* conversation? What *exactly* did they talk about as they hid from God? I personally don't think they talked about it. It makes much more sense that they hid separately, in isolation, just like we do now. Regardless of the blame that was thrown around, or the silence that comes from sin, it seems that we have all learned how to hide like Adam and Eve.

It's not just hiding that's the problem. It's what we do while we hide as well. It's been my experience that we tend to create something while we hide. Adam not only came up with a creative story to blame his wife, but he also physically created some type of makeshift underwear with fig leaves.

Trigger #6: Concealment

Unfortunately, you and I tend to create something much less noticeable. We create a false persona and personality.[70] We try to protect ourselves by covering up and pretending to be someone that we're not. I created an alter-ego of myself. My ego drove me to focus on my appearance, getting into shape and trying anything to have more hair! Needless to say, none of those ego-driven activities worked for long. I thought I could hide my pain through my exterior façade. I was pretending to be someone else because I wanted to conceal all my weaknesses and imperfections.

I was trying to protect myself from myself because I falsely believed that no one else would protect me. We hide because we've been abandoned, hurt, and rejected by too many people. We believe the lie that it's just easier to be alone. Fear from being found out will always drive us to hide. But the apostle John reminds us in 1 John 4:18 (ESV), **"There is no fear in love, but perfect love casts out fear. For fear has to do with punishment, and whoever fears has not been perfected in love."**[71]

Perfect love happens in a safe, Christ-centered community. Isolation never brings forth love, only fear. We hide because we don't want anyone to find out who we really are, and we conceal our behavior because of shame. We falsely believe that if people found out about the "real me," they wouldn't be our friend. We tell ourselves, "I'm too messed up. I've made too many mistakes and hurt too many people." I also hide because I think that it's up to me to fix me. It's one thing to go to the "self-help" section of a bookstore and learn how to prepare a budget. It's entirely different to try and fix your "addiction." The problem is that no matter how hard you try, you can't fix you.

Admitting to yourself that you're the problem is a giant step forward. Think about it—you're the one that got yourself into this mess in first place. Have you noticed that the more you try to fix yourself,

---

70 Turner, Mike. "Immersion Workshop Series." Workshop, Seven Places Ministries, Phoenix, January 2014.
71 *The Holy Bible: English Standard Version*. Wheaton: Standard Bible Society, 2016.

the messier life gets? This is a nasty side effect from hiding. Hiding prevents us from not dealing with the core issue—sin.

Sin is why secular counseling and programs don't work. They only give the illusion of healing through advice that produces short-term behavioral change. The *DSM* (*Diagnostic and Statistical Manual of Mental Disorders*) is the bible for secular counseling. The problem is that the *DSM* doesn't and will never define and treat the real problem—sin.

THE REAL PROBLEM

At this point in the spiral, we have a problem. The problem is that we have gone through six triggers and still believe that we haven't done anything wrong. Yes, I'm in hiding and about to act out in sin; but at this point, I'm telling myself that I haven't done anything wrong... *yet*.

If they "haven't done anything wrong," then most Christians will deal only with their acting out because it's the acting out that's wrong. No, no, no! The acting out is *not* the only thing that is wrong. ALL OF THIS IS WRONG.

John 3:19b reads, **"God's light came into the world, but people loved the darkness more than the light, for their actions were evil."** This is true of sin. Hiding moves us away from God and away from others to commit the sin. It is often said that the Bible will keep you from sin, but sin will also keep you from the Bible.

It's extremely important to understand that what you're about to do *must* be done in hiding. When you *choose* to hide, you're moments away from acting out in sin but, at the same time, wanting to conceal everything about it. Keep in mind that it's never too late to exit the spiral by fleeing, confessing, and/or praying. When you choose to trust somebody at *any* of these trigger points, the power of that sin is broken. Sin will *always* be broken when it's brought into the light.

Trigger #6: Concealment

BUT I DID CONFESS SIN!

Some of you may be thinking, *I am confessing my sin, but these Scriptures are not working!* If you find yourself in a cycle of sin/confess, sin/confess and are not experiencing any kind of momentum towards healing, there are several possibilities that are keeping you in bondage:

1. There has been little or no effort toward obedience. Confession and prayer are just halfhearted habits. Obedience is a sign of your love for God. The consequences have not become severe enough for *true* repentance. Most people start to change only when they have to.
2. There's a good possibility that you're confessing the wrong sin. You may be "apologizing" for sin, but not confessing to God that you *love* the pleasure that your sin of pornography brings.

LAMENT AND REPENT

Repentance requires that you completely abandon your old life—after all, you are dead to it. That's very different from confession. Confession is admitting your sin and guilt before God and others. Unfortunately, for many of us, confession is just lip service. The prophet Jeremiah introduces us to a new concept called *lamenting*. Lamenting is associated with a song of mourning and sorrow. It's where we make an appeal to overcome this calamity that we find ourselves in.

Jeremiah writes in Lamentations 2:18-19, **"Cry aloud before the Lord, O walls of beautiful Jerusalem! Let your tears flow like a river day and night. Give yourselves no rest; give your eyes no relief. Rise during the night and cry out. Pour out your hearts like water to the Lord. Lift up your hands to him in prayer, pleading for your children, for in every street they are faint with hunger."** Have you ever lamented over your sexual sin? Have you ever cried out before the Lord so much that your tears flowed like a river day after day and night after night?

The prophet Joel calls us to repentance in Joel 2:12-13, *"That is why the Lord says, 'Turn to me now, while there is time. Give me your hearts. Come with fasting, weeping, and mourning. Don't tear your clothing in your grief, but tear your hearts instead.' Return to the Lord your God, for he is merciful and compassionate, slow to get angry and filled with unfailing love. He is eager to relent and not punish."* Repentance is not about perfection, but persistence. Repentance allows you to grieve.

Your sin angers you. It makes you disgusted with yourself. It motivates you to do *whatever it takes* to make things right—*no matter the cost to you*. Ultimately, you start to hate your sin. If you haven't gone through these emotions, I'm guessing you have been only confessing (apologizing) your sin and have never truly repented. Going through the process of repentance reveals the kind of person you really are. We prove our thankfulness for God's forgiveness by taking action and being pro-active in choosing not to participate in looking at any more pornography.

The Lord Jesus Christ loves you more than you will ever understand (Jn. 3:16). He knows you better than you know yourself (Ps. 139:13, Jer. 1:5). He knows when you get up and sit down (Ps. 139:2). He knows every thought and every desire of your heart (Ps. 139:2). You will not scare or shock Him in any way.

I would like to encourage you to go through this process of repentance. The prophet Joel gives us the outline by fasting, weeping, and mourning. I would encourage you to spend the rest of today in prayer and start fasting tomorrow. Fasting is an excellent reminder of the seriousness of your sin. Choose to eat one meal a day for the next forty days. When your body cries out for food, pray! Ask the Lord to accept your fasting as a sign of repentance.

You can also begin right now by praying the following prayer.

> Father, I must confess to You that I love the pleasure that my pornography brings. In fact, I love it more than I love You. I love it more than I love people. That's why I continue to rebel

Trigger #6: Concealment

and run from You. I'm worshipping the creature instead of You, my Creator.

Father, please forgive me for taking Your grace and mercy for granted. Please humble me. Please take everything away from me, so I will stop making intentional choices that harm other people. Please do whatever it takes in my life to mold me into the man (or woman) you have destined me to be. Please change me no matter the cost to me. In Jesus' Name, Amen.

Lastly, there is a godly way to hide and conceal. By praying the prayer above, you have made the choice of doing just that. There is a way to hide God's Word in your heart through confession, lamenting, and repenting. As you walk this journey, you'll notice that this is not a one-time event, but rather something that we do on a daily, and sometimes hourly, basis.

Psalm 32:7 (ESV)—*"You are a hiding place for me; you preserve me from trouble; you surround me with shouts of deliverance."*[72]

Psalm 119:114 (ESV)—*"You are my hiding place and my shield; I hope in your word."*[73]

Matthew 13:44—*"The kingdom of heaven is like treasure hidden in a field, which a man found and covered up. Then in his joy he goes and sells all that he has and buys that field."*[74]

Colossians 3:2-4—*"Set your minds on things that are above, not on things that are on earth. For you have died, and your life is hidden with Christ in God. When Christ who is your life appears, then you also will appear with him in glory."*

When we learn how to seek for that treasure and realize that our lives are indeed hidden with Christ in God, there is no greater peace. It is a peace that surpasses our understanding (Phil. 4:7).

---

72 *The Holy Bible: English Standard Version.* Wheaton: Standard Bible Society, 2016.
73 Ibid.
74 Ibid.

CHAPTER 9

TRIGGER #7: ACTING OUT IN SIN

THE TEXT MESSAGE READ, "CALL me ASAP." My wife is not one to send urgent texts, so I called her immediately. Amy answered in a somber voice, "There's a problem with our foster care application, and DCS (Department of Child Safety) is asking to speak with you right away." She was on the verge of tears.

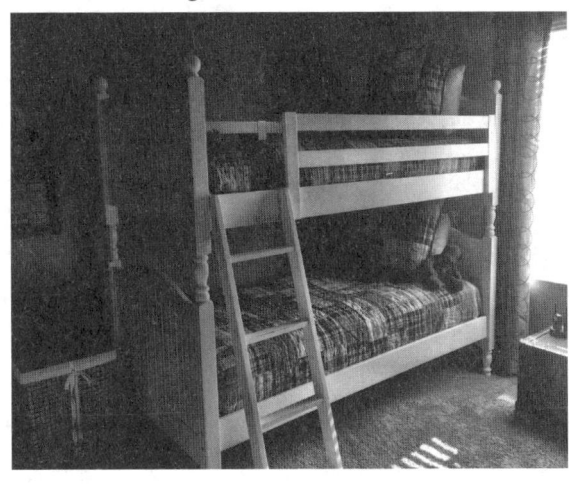

We had spent the last ten months preparing to bring foster children into our home. We had attended all the classes, filled out all the paperwork, and gone through multiple interviews. We completely converted our home-office into a second bedroom with bunk beds, dressers, toys, stuffed animals, and more. We had been praying and planning on caring for two brothers between the ages of five and eleven. DCS said that it's difficult to find a home that will accept two brothers at the same time. They prefer to keep siblings together through this traumatic event if at all possible.

I called DCS. In reviewing our file, they had become concerned about the sexual abuse that I had experienced while I was a child. They also wanted "proof" from a licensed, state-approved counselor that I had been "cured" from my own pornography addiction. They never said that I wasn't a "safe" person around children, but they certainly implied it. This insinuation leveled me. I screamed at myself, *They actually believe that I'm a threat to children!*

I never visited a licensed counselor during my "addiction years." I was (in DCS' words) "cured" by the Gospel through Jesus Christ. It's that simple. I met Jesus Christ and chose to obey and follow Him. My freedom has come from God packaging His Word into the very material that you are reading now. I explained in great detail that teaching and training God's design for sex, marriage, and the family were my life's work because of my past. Regardless, they questioned more of my background and theological training. They asked for proof, requesting certification after certification. I had to explain that my "pornography addiction" didn't involve children whatsoever. Nevertheless, after several more conference calls with DCS, we had to withdraw our foster care application. Ultimately, the "religious" counseling I had received was deemed invalid because it wasn't licensed by the government.

Needless to say, that was a tough day. I understand their view and applaud DCS for the tough decisions that they must make on a daily basis. It took us months to even think about it, but we had no choice but to tear down the boys' room. It felt like we had lost these children without even meeting them. This experience was just as painful as when Amy had a miscarriage during our first year of marriage.

I must admit—I didn't see that conversation coming. It hit me so hard that it threw me into a situational depression. The consequences of my sin still seem to point and laugh—not just at me but at my wife and foster children as well. There is a reality to all of my past sin that I'm still uncomfortable thinking about. It's the reality that I'll never be a father. Yes, indeed, my friend, the consequences of acting out in sin are weighty.

ACTING OUT IN SIN

Trigger #7 is Acting Out in Sin. This is the actual behavior of the sin itself. It's the way that you choose to finally satisfy your lust. At this point in the spiral, you become drunk with lust. You are intoxicated with entitlement and deserve sexual satisfaction. The seduction of the promised pleasure simply prevents any rational, God-fearing behavior.

A lot of books that are written on recovery or addiction *start* with acting out. They begin by teaching people how to manage sin or how not to sin. The problem, however, is that you've already blown through six opportunities where you could have exited the sex spiral through fleeing, confessing, and/or praying.

By the time you get to Trigger #7, it's far too late for sin management. In fact, there is no such thing. By this trigger, so much has built up—unhealthy thoughts, temptation, resistance, rationalization, concealment—that there is *no way* you are managing this spiral! In fact, when that thought crosses your mind, you have trusted in the weakest person on earth—yourself.

At this trigger, you can't even think through the lust to imagine the consequences. It's impossible. Plus, truth be told, you don't even care. All you can focus on is the promised pleasure of the sin itself. During this trigger, nothing—and I mean *nothing*—but pleasure is more important.

Once we make the conscious and willful decision to sin and then regretfully look back at what we have just done, it's entirely too late. The consequences *are* coming. There is no way to avoid them.

BECAUSE YOU HAVE DONE THIS

In Genesis 3:11-23, we read about eight consequences that not only happened to Adam and Eve but also impacted God Himself, along with the rest of mankind. Let's look at them below:

"Who told you that you were naked?" the Lord God asked. "Have you eaten from the tree whose fruit I commanded you not to eat?"

The man replied, "It was the woman you gave me who gave me the fruit, and I ate it."

Then the Lord God asked the woman, "What have you done?"

"The serpent deceived me," she replied. "That's why I ate it."

Then the Lord God said to the serpent, "Because you have done this, you are cursed more than all animals, domestic and wild. You will crawl on your belly, groveling in the dust as long as you live **(Consequence #1)**.

And I will cause hostility between you and the woman **(Consequence #2)**, and between your offspring and her offspring **(Consequence #3)**. He will strike your head, and you will strike his heel."

Then He said to the woman, "I will sharpen the pain of your pregnancy, and in pain you will give birth **(Consequence #4)**. And you will desire to control your husband **(Consequence #5)**, but he will rule over you" **(Consequence #6)**.

And to the man he said, "Since you listened to your wife and ate from the tree whose fruit I commanded you not to eat, the ground is cursed because of you **(Consequence #7)**. All your life you will struggle to scratch a living from it.

It will grow thorns and thistles for you, though you will eat of its grains.

Trigger #7: Acting Out in Sin

By the sweat of your brow will you have food to eat until you return to the ground from which you were made. For you were made from dust, and to dust you will return."

Then the man—Adam—named his wife Eve, because she would be the mother of all who live.

And the Lord God made clothing from animal skins for Adam and his wife.

Then the Lord God said, "Look, the human beings have become like us, knowing both good and evil. What if they reach out, take fruit from the tree of life, and eat it? Then they will live forever!"

So the Lord God banished them from the Garden of Eden **(Consequence #8)**, and he sent Adam out to cultivate the ground from which he had been made.

WELCOME TO REALITY

Uncontrollable consequences have now been set in motion due to acting out—just as they were for Adam. Have you ever seen the absolute power and authority of a tsunami wave? If you haven't, visit YouTube to get the full picture of its wrath. A tsunami happens when the sea floor shifts, which then causes the water above to cause a massive series of waves. It's like an underwater earthquake. These waves now have no choice but to devastate everything in their path.

It's not just the initial tsunami wave that causes damage either. Once the wave devastates everything in its path, the water then pulls that wreckage back out into the ocean. Another wave will then come inland—this time with the previous wreckage, which causes even more damage. This back and forth process could take place for hours.

Habitual sin with pornography is like a tsunami wave. Once you act out, it's like the proverbial "ocean floor" being disrupted, catapulting these tsunami waves of consequences into your life. The problem that we have at this point is misunderstanding God's grace. Because of God's grace, He gives us lots of time (years and even decades) to humble ourselves through confession and repentance. However, when consequences don't seem to show up, we tend to believe that all is well. Fortunately, God loves you too much not to be disciplined.

The Bible speaks many times about the consequences that sin brings.

- James 1:15—*"These desires give birth to sinful actions. And when sin is allowed to grow, it gives birth to death."*
- Romans 6:23a—*"For the wages of sin is death."*
- Proverbs 28:26 (ESV)—*"Whoever trusts in his own mind is a fool, but he who walks in wisdom will be delivered."*[75]

It's impossible to manage the pleasure of sin and absurd to think that we can manipulate the consequences of it.

- Galatians 6:7-8—*"Don't be misled—you cannot mock the justice of God. You will always harvest what you plant. Those who live only to satisfy their own sinful nature will harvest decay and death from that sinful nature. But those who live to please the Spirit will harvest everlasting life from the Spirit."*

"ADDICT" OR SINNER

You may or may not be a porn or sex "addict." The reality is that it doesn't matter because you are a sinner—just like me. The apostle Paul tells us in Romans 3:23, *"For everyone has sinned; we all fall short of God's glorious standard."* Now, keep in mind when dealing with

---

75 *The Holy Bible: English Standard Version.* Wheaton: Standard Bible Society, 2016.

sexual sin, that you're dealing with a sin issue first and a physiological and psychological issue second.

Think about this—Jesus stepped off His throne in heaven; was born of a virgin; lived a perfect, sinless life; and was humiliated, beaten, and murdered *because* of our sin. He also chose to raise Himself from the dead, walk out of His own grave, and show Himself to hundreds of people to prove that He was, indeed, God. Then He ascended back into heaven from where He came and now sits at the right hand of His Father, reigning and ruling the entire universe. If Jesus did all of that for the sole purpose of *forgiving* you, is it possible that He can also *free* you from your propensity toward lust? Of course. When we get our eyes off our sin and onto our Savior, everything changes.

The issue is understanding how forgiveness and freedom work. The forgiveness of Christ was based solely on His love toward you. You didn't do *anything* to receive it. By God's grace, He chose you to be His child. The apostle Paul reminds us in Romans 5:6-8, **"When we were utterly helpless, Christ came at just the right time and died for us sinners. Now, most people would not be willing to die for an upright person, though someone might perhaps be willing to die for a person who is especially good. But God showed his great love for us by sending Christ to die for us while we were still sinners."** In other words, you didn't do a single thing to be forgiven by Jesus Christ. He did *all* the work for you. He *chose* to love you!

Now, it doesn't work the same way with breaking free from a habitual sin like pornography. Learning how to be free in your forgiveness takes a tremendous amount of cooperation on your end. Please don't hear what I didn't say. I didn't say that you have the ability to do this on your own. Nope, this kind of freedom is based on the Lord's terms. You must now cooperate *with* the power of the Holy Spirit who dwells in you. Just as Jesus gave His disciples an option to follow Him, you now have a choice to follow Him as well.[76]

---

[76] There are over twenty references to "Follow Me" in the Gospels.

Many of us believe that if God forgave our sin by doing all the work, then He will do all the work in our "addiction" as well. That's not true either. There is a colossal difference between being forgiven by Christ (justifiable salvation) and being free in Christ (progressive sanctification). Let's take a look.

CUT IT OFF OR CUT IT OUT

If your hand causes you to sin, cut it off. It's better to enter eternal life with only one hand than to go into the unquenchable fires of hell with two hands. If your foot causes you to sin, cut it off. It's better to enter eternal life with only one foot than to be thrown into hell with two feet. And if your eye causes you to sin, gouge it out. It's better to enter the Kingdom of God with only one eye than to have two eyes and be thrown into hell, "where the maggots never die and the fire never goes out." For everyone will be tested with fire (Mk. 9:43-49).

You have heard the commandment that says, "You must not commit adultery." But I say, anyone who even looks at a woman with lust has already committed adultery with her in his heart. So if your eye—even your good eye—causes you to lust, gouge it out and throw it away. It is better for you to lose one part of your body than for your whole body to be thrown into hell. And if your hand—even your stronger hand—causes you to sin, cut it off and throw it away. It is better for you to lose one part of your body than for your whole body to be thrown into hell (Matt. 5:27-30).

What's the point? Is Jesus exaggerating to get our attention, or is He being literal? Let's think about this. If you were to gouge out your eye, wouldn't you still be able to sin with the other? If you gouged out *both*

Trigger #7: Acting Out in Sin

eyes, wouldn't you still be able to lust through the fantasies that you can conjure up in the library of your mind? If you cut off your hand to keep from sinning, wouldn't you still be able to sin with the other? I believe Jesus is exaggerating to make a point that most of us completely ignore. *We must be willing to do whatever it takes—no matter the cost to me—to stop sinning.* Sin is a heart issue (Lk. 6:43-45). In other words, it's an internal, spiritual reality that is demonstrated by our external behavior.

YOUR BRAIN ON PORN

Let's now discuss the physiological side of pornography. Please allow me to add a disclaimer before we begin. Although I will be using medical terminology to give a simple overview of what happens to the male brain during this trigger, the terminology may still surprise or shock you. Please know that is not my intent. My purpose is to be clear about why the pleasure of sex is addictive from a medical perspective.

HERE'S THE DEAL

So, what happens when men act out? In other words, what happens during masturbation and ejaculation? Well, believe it or not, our brains have a lot more to do with sex than any other body part. In its simplest form, there's stimulation that comes from the spinal cord that goes to the reward circuitry part of the brain. It's known as "the pleasure center." When there's ejaculation, there's a release of dopamine. This shuts down a part of the brain called the "amygdala." The amygdala is the emotional and fear center in the brain. Why is that important? An orgasm is associated with an *absence* of fear. Many men experience a supernatural-type of freedom from worry. Ultimately, ejaculation makes us temporarily worry free. That is why we take such huge risks with sexual sin. Many risk their marriage, job, children, STDs, and dozens of other consequences—all or in part to be *temporarily worry-free*. For more information on how porn impacts the brain, I would suggest *Wired for Intimacy: How Pornography Hijacks the Male Brain* by William Struthers.[77]

It's amazing that scientists can tell us how the brain functions in great detail. What they can't tell us, however, is what we're actually thinking. They can tell us how much adrenaline and dopamine have gone through our brain, but they can't tell us the lustful thought that caused it. This is why the apostle Paul writes in Romans 12:2, **"Don't copy the behavior and customs of this world, <u>but let God transform you into a new person by changing the way you think.</u> Then you will learn to know God's will for you, which is good and pleasing and perfect"** (emphasis mine).

After you have acted out in sin, what happens next? You will most likely go back into hiding, but this time it directly impacts those that love you the most. It's called *relational withdraw*, and it's our next trigger.

---

[77] Struthers, William. *Wired for Intimacy: How Pornography Hijacks the Male Brain*. Downers Grove: Intervarsity Press, 2010.

CHAPTER 10

TRIGGER #8: RELATIONAL WITHDRAW

RELATIONAL WITHDRAWAL IS AN IMMEDIATE effect of acting out. When I choose to act out in sin, something begins to happen to me relationally *and* spiritually. I have not only been blatantly disobedient to the Lord, but I have violated my own conscience. I have broken my own set of guardrails for morality.

The reason I feel guilty after acting out in sin is because my own conscience condemns me. Also, the Holy Spirit uses healthy guilt to urge me to confess my sin. If I don't move toward God and others, I will remove myself from all relationships. I once again am trying to protect myself, but by doing so, I end up avoiding the very people that love and care for me most.

This is where we see our outward effects of shame on other people. This is where internal, shameful thoughts (Trigger #2) begin to reveal themselves with external consequences. Internal thoughts can't stay internal. They will manifest themselves outwardly in one way or another over time.

Once I've withdrawn, unhealthy guilt and shame begin to thrive like cockroaches in the dark. Do you remember our definition of "shame"? Shame is the disgraceful feeling existing from sin, failure, public exposure, and/or dishonor. It's a painful emotion and feeling because I've done something dishonorable or something dishonorable has been done to me. We think, *Since my behavior is a disgrace, I must be a disgrace.* Shame is not that I've done something stupid; shame says that I *am* stupid. Shame is not that I've made a mistake; shame screams that I *am* a mistake. I've done something dishonorable, therefore I *must be* dishonorable. My acting out in sin is disgusting, therefore *I'm a disgusting person*. Ultimately, shame is believing that I am my behavior and that I am powerless over my sin. These are all lies; but because I've withdrawn myself from the most important people in my life, my behavior convinces me that I don't like me; I don't like you; and I don't like God either. I falsely believe that because of what I've done (or what's been done to me), I'm unforgivable. If I falsely believe that I'm unforgivable, then I also falsely believe that I'm unlovable.

MORE HIDING

In Trigger #6 (Concealment), we learned that we will go into hiding right before we act out in sin. The same is also true *after* we commit the sin. The difference here is that because I've acted out in sin, my shame now demands more isolation.

My feelings and attitudes now move away from my family and friends. Shame (Trigger #2) forces me to distance myself from the very people who love and care for me the most. For example: While at work, you're distracted and unproductive. Because you're distracted and unproductive, you're becoming more and more irritable with colleagues, customers, or work itself. You may be physically present at work or with your family and friends, but you're not really there with them emotionally. Because you're really not there, the people who love you the most begin asking questions like, "You okay?" or "What's wrong?" These prying questions into your sin only fuel your shame, creating anger (Trigger #11).

BUT I DON'T HAVE ANY FRIENDS

Chad was a good-looking, slender, middle-aged man in his fifties. He owned and operated a successful business that didn't need much oversight. He told me he was bored a lot of the time. This boredom got him into trouble with pornography. As he was wrestling with God and trying not to argue with his wife one day, she noticed his boredom and told him to call a friend and go play golf. He liked the idea and

Trigger #8: Relational Withdraw

was thinking of who he could call. He then told me, "I don't have any friends to even go play golf with! How pathetic is that?"

If you don't have any friends like Chad, then there is a good chance that your sin has become your "friend." To have friends, we must first be friends to others. Has pornography become your friend? Have strip clubs and massage parlors become your community?

One question I ask in our groups is, "Tell me about your quiet time with the Lord. What does that look like?" Being involved in a habitual sin like pornography prevents a longing to be with the Lord. The quietness of the quiet time seems to be deafening, and the thought of approaching the Lord in your current condition is terrifying (as it should be). After this question, the cold, paralyzing reality begins to set in—if we spend time with people and the things that we love and I'm spending more time with pornography than with God, then I love my porn more than God.

"SHE'LL LEAVE ME"

Todd confessed to me that after three months of being sexually sober, he had "slipped up" last night. I could see the frustration on his face. He was mad at himself. He had been going through this spiral off and on for years.

I asked him, "Did you tell your wife?"

He looked at me in complete terror, "NO! She'll leave me if I do."

"How do you know that?" I asked.

Todd snapped back, "I just do, okay?"

"No, you don't, Todd," I replied. "You don't know what tomorrow will bring (Jas. 4:14-16). You think you have control over this, but you don't have control over anything. If you did, your life wouldn't be such a mess right now, would it?"

Todd's face flushed with anger at this point. His eyes turned dark, trying to intimidate me.

I continued, "You're talking to me as if I'm the villain, but I'm simply trying to love you. Sure, you're sorry, but who isn't? Are you sorry enough to *change*? Are you *mad enough* to change? If you are, then go home and confess your sin to your wife."

Many times, we think we have repented, when we have not. The reason for this is our unwillingness to bring our sin out into the light to others. If we don't confess our sin to our spouse and trusted friends, healing cannot and will not take place (Jas. 5:16). The result is a continued state of relational withdraw from God.

True repentance is facing those who have been affected by your sin and accepting full responsibility for the upcoming consequences without Justification (Trigger #9) or Blame (Trigger #10). Todd was still unwilling to do this after several years of being with me in the ministry. That's why I took the position I did. I loved him too much to allow him to wallow in his sin and at the same time continue to emotionally abuse his family.

If Todd were to face his wife and move toward a healthy relationship, he could have moved toward restoration and healing. Compulsive and unrepentant people don't move toward those things. Can you see how Todd was not repentant—no matter how mad he was at himself? He ultimately still loved his sin too much and left the very people who were trying to help. Unrepentant people say "I'm sorry"— sometimes with tears—but slowly move back into isolation and into the sex spiral.

True repentance produces transparency, along with an eagerness to make amends. True repentance brings a spirit of renewed joy and a new confidence in God. It brings peacefulness in our lives, an intimacy with God, and joy in His presence.

Remember the tsunami wave? It's coming for Todd. This is what habitual sin does. It forces us to do the very opposite of what we need to do. What Todd failed to realize is that confession is a way to lower the threshold of pain before the tsunami wave hits his shore.

Trigger #8: Relational Withdraw

SHAME REVISITED

At this point in *The Sex Spiral*, you probably don't like yourself. You shut down. You're numb and angry. You have your mask on. You're faking it, but you kid yourself when you think that the charade is working. However, your family and friends know something is wrong. Everything is not "fine." They feel your emotional and spiritual absence, even though you're physically present, but they can't get into your shame. They can't get into your mind. They can guess at what the problem is, but they can't go there because you won't let them in.

THE CURE

How do you remedy the situation? You must replace the lies with God's truth. I have found that the Word of God is best used when spoken *out loud*. There is power in the spoken word of the Lord. After all, God spoke the world into existence (Gen. 1:3-26), and Jesus spoke Lazarus' name for him to rise from the dead (Jn. 11:43).

Read the verse below out loud over and over with confidence.

That is why the Lord says, "Turn to me now, while there is time. Give me your hearts. Come with fasting, weeping, and mourning. Don't tear your clothing in your grief, but tear your hearts instead." Return to the Lord your God, for he is merciful and compassionate, slow to get angry and filled with unfailing love. He is eager to relent and not punish (Joel 2:12-13).

Isn't that amazing? God is saying, "Look, I know what you've done, and I'm telling you that *even now*, return to Me, and I will forgive you! I will free you!" But what happens if we don't repent?

- Acts 17:30—**"God overlooked people's ignorance about these things in earlier times, but now he commands everyone everywhere to repent of their sins and turn to him."**

- Romans 2:4—*"Don't you see how wonderfully kind, tolerant, and patient God is with you? Does this mean nothing to you? Can't you see that his kindness is intended to turn you from your sin?"*

In other words, God's kindness and grace is an opportunity for you to repent. The opportunity also comes with a deadline. His kindness is not intended for you, so you can keep on sinning.

- Romans 6:1-2—*"Well then, should we keep on sinning so that God can show us more and more of his wonderful grace? Of course not! Since we have died to sin, how can we continue to live in it?"*

What if you're no longer bothered by your sin and behavior? Now this is where life gets serious.

Jesus said in Matthew 7:21-23:

> *Not everyone who calls out to me, "Lord! Lord!" will enter the Kingdom of Heaven. Only those who actually do the will of my Father in heaven will enter. On judgment day many will say to me, "Lord! Lord! We prophesied in your name and cast out demons in your name and performed many miracles in your name." But I will reply, "I never knew you. Get away from me, you who break God's laws."*

But what if you are reading this book, desperately searching for answers as to why you continue to behave in this way? The apostle Paul writes in Philippians 2:12-13, *"Dear friends, you always followed my instructions when I was with you. And now that I am away, it is even more important. Work hard to show the results of your salvation, obeying God with deep reverence and fear. For God is working in you, giving you the desire and the power to do what pleases him."*

Matthew 3:8 tells us, *"Prove by the way you live that you have repented of your sins and turned to God."* For many people, confession, and repentance are something they do with God. They say, "I really mean it this time, God. I promise that I won't do it again!" However, the promise is between only God and you. When you make this deal with God, you need to check yourself. You need to ask, "If I'm serious about change, why am I hesitating or even refusing to tell someone else?" Remember Todd's story?

FALSE HOPE

False repentance produces a false hope of change. In other words, saying, "I'm sorry" doesn't really do anything. Most wives that have been abused by their husband's porn use hate those two words with a passion. Why? Because false repentance produces hopelessness (Trigger #12). As men, we tend to believe that knowledge is all we need to change. The reality is that you don't need the knowledge in this book to change. Knowledge can produce a false hope because knowledge, by itself, does not yield a relationship with God. Just because you read an autobiography of someone you admire, that doesn't mean you know him or her. You simply know about him or her.

When it comes to your relationship with Jesus, I'm guessing there were certain things that you did when you first became a Christian that you don't do now for a variety of reasons.[78]

Look at these different versions of Revelation 2:4-5:

"But I have this complaint against you. You don't love me or each other as you did at first! Look how far you have fallen! Turn back to me and do the works you did at first. If you don't repent, I will come and remove your lampstand from its place among the churches."

"But you walked away from your first love—why? What's going on with you, anyway? Do you have any idea how far you've fallen? A Lucifer fall! Turn back! Recover your dear early love. No time to waste, for I'm well on my way to removing your light from the golden circle" (The Message).[79]

---

78 Weiss, Dr. Doug. *Clean: A Proven Plan for Men Committed to Sexual Integrity.* Nashville: Thomas Nelson, 2013.
79 Peterson, Eugene H. *The Message: The Bible in Contemporary Language.* Colorado Springs: NavPress, 2005.

"However, I have this against you: you have abandoned your first love. Do you remember what it was like before you fell? It's time to rethink and change your ways; go back to how you first acted. However, if you do not return, I will come quickly and personally remove your lampstand from its place" (The Voice).[80]

Think back to the time when you felt the closest to the Lord. What were the specific things that you were doing during that time? Jesus tells you very plainly that you have been distracted with things that don't matter. These distractions in your life have tripped you up. Yes, you have fallen, and it is a mighty fall indeed. But all is not lost. Jesus is literally telling you to "turn back to Me and do the works you did at first."

If you choose not to do the works you did at first, you'll continue down the next layer in the sex spiral. Let's move to Trigger #9—Justification.

---

80 Ecclesia Bible Society, *The Voice*, Nashville, Thomas Nelson, 2012.

CHAPTER 11

TRIGGER #9: JUSTIFICATION

ON JANUARY 26, 1998, PRESIDENT Bill Clinton said, "I want to say one thing to the American people. I want you to listen to me. I'm going to say this again. I did not have sexual relations with that woman—Miss Lewinsky. I never told anybody to lie, not a single time. Never."[81] Why did President Clinton have to say this to the American people? Robert Bennett (President Clinton's attorney) had stated that there "is" no sexual relationship between Bill Clinton and Monica Lewinsky. President Clinton was then asked for further clarification by the Grand Jury on Mr. Bennett's statement. Below is a transcript of what President Clinton said verbatim.

> It depends on what the meaning of the word "is" is. If the—if he—if "is" means "is" and "never has been" . . . that is not—that is one thing. If it means "there is none," that was a completely true statement. Now, if someone had asked me on that day, are you having any kind of sexual relations with Ms. Lewinsky, that is, asked me a question in the present tense, I would have said no. And it would have been completely true."[82]

---

81 *The Washington Post*. "What Clinton Said." WashingtonPost.com. http://www.washingtonpost.com/wp-srv/politics/special/clinton/stories/whatclintonsaid.htm (accessed May 2017).
82 Miller, Jake. "15 Years Ago: Bill Clinton Historical Denial." CBS News. http://www.cbsnews.com/news/15-years-ago-bill-clintons-historic-denial/ (accessed January 26, 2013).

Welcome to Justification—Trigger #9. Justification is the acceptable reason we do something immoral. You are trying to prove that it was reasonable, essentially defending your position.

Now, please don't confuse justification with rationalization. Rationalization (Trigger #5) is the way of convincing yourself to engage in the sin. We rationalize what we are getting ready to do while we justify what we have just done.

THE MEANING OF THE WORD "IS"

Did you believe President Clinton and his statement about not having sexual relations with Monica Lewinsky? Did his explanation of the word "is" make any sense to you? If it didn't, that's okay. It didn't make sense to anyone *but* President Clinton himself. That's the power of justification. It makes sense only to the people caught in the sin. For the rest of us listening, the lies are laughably pathetic. The unfortunate reality, however, is that we *really believe* what we are saying is true. It's like a new chapter of *The Emperor's New Clothes*.

An Apology

Seven months later, on August 31, 1998, President Clinton apologized to the American people. He said:

> This afternoon in this room, from this chair, I testified before the Office of Independent Counsel and the Grand Jury.
>
> I answered their questions truthfully, including questions about my private life, questions no American citizen would ever want to answer. Still, I must take complete responsibility for all my actions, both public and private. And that is why I am speaking to you tonight.
>
> As you know, in a deposition in January, I was asked questions about my relationship with Monica Lewinsky. While my answers were legally accurate, I did not volunteer information. Indeed, I did have a relationship with Miss Lewinsky

Trigger #9: Justification

that was not appropriate. In fact, it was wrong. It constituted a critical lapse in judgment and a personal failure on my part for which I am solely and completely responsible.

But I told the Grand Jury today and I say to you now that at no time did I ask anyone to lie, to hide or destroy evidence or to take any other unlawful action.

I know that my public comments and my silence about this matter gave a false impression. I misled people, including even my wife. I deeply regret that.

I can only tell you I was motivated by many factors. First, by a desire to protect myself from the embarrassment of my own conduct. I was also very concerned about protecting my family. The fact that these questions were being asked in a politically inspired lawsuit, which has since been dismissed, was a consideration, too.

The independent counsel investigation moved on to my staff and friends, then into my private life. And now the investigation itself is under investigation. This has gone on too long, cost too much and hurt too many innocent people.

Now, this matter is between me, the two people I love most—my wife and our daughter—and our God. I must put it right, and I am prepared to do whatever it takes to do so. Nothing is more important to me personally. But it is private, and I intend to reclaim my family life for my family. It's nobody's business but ours.

Even presidents have private lives. It is time to stop the pursuit of personal destruction and the prying into private lives and get on with our national life.

Our country has been distracted by this matter for too long, and I take my responsibility for my part in all of this. That is all I can do. Now it is time—in fact, it is past time—to move on. We have important work to do—real opportunities to seize, real problems to solve, real security matters to face.

And so tonight, I ask you to turn away from the spectacle of the past seven months, to repair the fabric of our national discourse, and to return our attention to all the challenges and all the promise of the next American century.[83]

From The White House

In 1998, as a result of issues surrounding personal indiscretions with a young woman—a White House intern—Clinton was the second U.S. president to be impeached by the House of Representatives. He was tried in the Senate and found not guilty of the charges brought against him. He apologized to the nation for his actions and continued to have unprecedented popular approval ratings for his job as president.[84]

PAUSE

It's easy to pick on President Clinton, but let's focus on us now. We are all rationalizers (Trigger #5); we are also justifiers and minimizers. It makes no sense to people listening, but we always have an excuse for our sin, don't we? We always have an absurd answer, but the answer makes sense to us because we are caught in this spiral.

Why do we always have an excuse? President Clinton gave this answer twice in his apology. Justification is our attempt at self-protection. We justify our behavior because we don't want to face the reality of what we've actually done. At this point, we may see how silly or stupid the rationalization we gave ourselves was to commit the sin, but we

---

83 Ibid.
84 Freidel, Frank and Hugh Sidey. *The Presidents of the United States of America*. Scala Publishers, 2006.

Trigger #9: Justification

usually won't admit it. We force ourselves to believe it, so we go on the defensive. It puts us on our heels. It tells our family and friends that we are refusing to own our behavior. There's a difference between an apology and an admission of sin. Apologies acknowledge a mistake, while an admission of sin is a confession of moral wrongdoing.

When we justify our sin, we tend to talk too much. When we talk too much, it all becomes nonsense. The half-brother of Jesus, James, has a lot to say about talking. He speaks specifically about how dangerous our tongue is. Below is an excerpt from James 3:2-12. I've added commentary to show us the seriousness of justification.

- *"Indeed, we all make many mistakes. For if we could control our tongues, we would be perfect and could also control ourselves in every other way"* (v. 2).

In other words, unless we stop making excuses for our sin, we will continue to be a slave to it. Once we begin the self-control of closing our mouths, the self-control of our behavior follows.

- *"We can make a large horse go wherever we want by means of a small bit in its mouth. And a small rudder makes a huge ship turn wherever the pilot chooses to go, even though the winds are strong. In the same way, the tongue is a small thing that makes grand speeches"* (vv. 3-5a).

Wasn't that a grand speech by President Clinton? Did you believe him? How about the apologies from pro golfer Tiger Woods or politician Anthony Weiner? More importantly, does your spouse, friend, and/or boss believe *your* grand speeches?

- *"But a tiny spark can set a great forest on fire. And among all the parts of the body, the tongue is a flame of fire. It is a whole world of wickedness, corrupting your entire body. It can set your whole life on fire, for it is set on fire by hell itself"* (vv. 5b-6).

Was it pornography that set your life on fire, or was it the lying, manipulating, and justifying of your sin?

- *"People can tame all kinds of animals, birds, reptiles, and fish, but no one can tame the tongue. It is restless and evil, full of deadly poison. Sometimes it praises our Lord and Father, and sometimes it curses those who have been made in the image of God. And so blessing and cursing come pouring out of the same mouth. Surely, my brothers and sisters, this is not right! Does a spring of water bubble out with both fresh water and bitter water? Does a fig tree produce olives, or a grapevine produce figs? No, and you can't draw fresh water from a salty spring"* (vv. 7-12).

There are many of us who attend church, listen to a sermon, and even raise our hands in praise during worship; but later that day, we use those same hands to click through pages and pages of pornographic images and videos. We use our words to ask God to bless us, while later in the day, we use other words to justify our sin. The apostle James is saying, *"Surely, my brothers and sisters, this is not right!"* (Jas. 3:10b).

AN EMOTIONAL BASEBALL BAT

Betty was in my office crying, her husband sitting right next to her, staring at the floor.

"I can forgive the pornography," Betty said. "But what I don't understand are the constant lies about it! Why can't you just tell me the truth?"

I waited for her husband, Jeff, to answer. He looked at me for help—as if I was going to swoop in and throw him a life preserver. After he couldn't take the silence anymore, he mumbled, "I . . . I . . . I don't know why. I don't know what to say."

Betty was exasperated. "WHAT? *You* don't know what to say? Jeff, you have an answer for EVERYTHING. And you know what's so stupid, Jeff? ME! I'm stupid for believing you."

Trigger #9: Justification

I asked Jeff to look at me. "Do you realize that every time you lie to your wife, every time you justify your sin, you are beating your wife with an emotional baseball bat?" Jeff frowned at my question.

"What would happen if you took a real baseball bat and hit your wife as hard as you could?" I asked.

Jeff responded, "I would never do that."

"I'm not saying you would, but what would happen if you did?" I asked.

"She would get hurt," Jeff answered apprehensively.

"How badly would she get hurt?" I inquired.

"Depends on where I hit her, I guess," Jeff murmured. "How about in the back, when she didn't see it coming?" I asked. Jeff looked back down at the floor.

"How about in her abdomen? Would you knock the wind out of her? Would you break her ribs?" I probed.

Silence filled the room. Betty's eyes continued to flow with a steady stream of tears.

"What about in the face, Jeff? What would happen if you swung a baseball bat and hit Betty in the face?"

Jeff looked at Betty and tried to grab her hand. She pulled back and crossed her arms. Jeff said, "Honey, I would never do that."

I pressed on further. "What about when she is lying on the floor, bleeding from the first set of blows, and you continue to strike her with the bat?"

Jeff still held firm. "Okay, that's enough. I said I would *never* do that."

"But you *are*, Jeff," I said, trying to shock him out of his complacency. "Every time you lie to Betty, you are hitting her with an *emotional* baseball bat. Can you see how devastated she is from years of abuse?"

"Abuse?" Jeff asked.

"Every time you lie to your wife, you are emotionally and spiritually *abusing* your wife," I said. "You have deeply wounded Betty's spirit with all your lies and deception. You have caused real hurt. This is real pain, Jeff. This is not a game. Your wife is showing symptoms of PTSD - post traumatic stress disorder."

I looked at Betty and asked, "Is that how you feel?"

She turned to Jeff and said, "That's *exactly* how I've felt—for years! I thought I was losing my mind trying to keep track of everything you've said because none of it made any sense, but you convinced me that it all made perfect sense! Jeff, I really thought I was going crazy."[85]

TALK IS CHEAP

It's one thing to look at pornography. It's another issue to lie, manipulate, and justify. Sin breeds more sin. Why do we lie and get tangled up in our lies? Just like President Clinton, we are trying to *protect* ourselves. Below is what God has to say about the weight of our words.

- Proverbs 10:19—*"Too much talk leads to sin. Be sensible and keep your mouth shut."*
- Proverbs 12:13—*"The wicked are trapped by their own words, but the godly escape such trouble."*
- Proverbs 18:21—*"The tongue can bring death or life; those who love to talk will reap the consequences."*
- Proverbs 21:23—*"Watch your tongue and keep your mouth shut, and you will stay out of trouble."*

THE SERIOUSNESS OF JUSTIFICATION

It's one thing to talk too much and justify your sin. It's another to justify your behavior and then use Scripture, out of context, to prove your position with your wife and children. Please hear me loud and clear—if you are doing this, you are *beating* your family down with God's Word, instead of lifting them up. When you do this, you are considered a false teacher. You preach a message you pretend to understand for the sole purpose of justifying your sin. This is where your sin

---

85 This manipulation technique is called Gaslighting.

gets really serious because the issue is no longer about pornography. It's about lying and scheming so that you can *continue* in pornography.

> But there were also false prophets in Israel, just as there will be false teachers among you. They will cleverly teach destructive heresies and even deny the Master who bought them. In this way, they will bring sudden destruction on themselves. Many will follow their evil teaching and shameful immorality. And because of these teachers, the way of truth will be slandered. In their greed they will make up clever lies to get hold of your money. But God condemned them long ago, and their destruction will not be delayed.
>
> He is especially hard on those who follow their own twisted sexual desire, and who despise authority. These people are proud and arrogant, daring even to scoff at supernatural beings without so much as trembling. But the angels, who are far greater in power and strength, do not dare to bring from the Lord a charge of blasphemy against those supernatural beings.
>
> These false teachers are like unthinking animals, creatures of instinct, born to be caught and destroyed. They scoff at things they do not understand, and like animals, they will be destroyed. Their destruction is their reward for the harm they have done. They love to indulge in evil pleasures in broad daylight. They are a disgrace and a stain among you. They delight in deception even as they eat with you in your fellowship meals. They commit adultery with their eyes, and their desire for sin is never satisfied. They lure unstable people into sin, and they are well trained in greed. They live under **God's curse** (2 Pet. 2:1-3; 10-14).

What you say matters. How you say it matters. Justification keeps you in the spiral. Repentance allows you to exit. We can do both with our tongues. One way to know that you are trapped in this trigger is by how much you are talking. If you can't answer a question with a simple yes or no, then there's a good chance you are justifying your behavior.

When you choose not to exit the sex spiral at this point, someone will always be the victim of your sin. Here we move down to the next layer, Trigger #10—Blame.

CHAPTER 12

TRIGGER #10: BLAME

AS YOU MOVE THROUGH THE trigger of justification, someone will always be blamed. In other words, someone is going to be the victim of your sin. It's usually someone you love like a spouse, child, other family member, or close friend. Blame is holding someone else responsible for *your* sinful actions. It's placing the responsibility of *your* behavior on someone else. Blame also allows *you* to move into a mindset of condemnation. *You* will criticize, reprimand, rebuke and find fault with others within this trigger because of *your* behavior.

Blame is the next natural cog in the wheel of sin. Think about it—just moments ago, in Trigger #9, you were emphatically justifying and excusing your behavior. So, if your behavior is not your fault, it must be someone else's. But, it is *your* fault, and that's why this chapter is so direct. Instead of you pointing your finger at someone else, you must realize that there are three other fingers pointing back at you when you blame someone else.

CHOICES

You have several choices when it comes to blame. First, you can confess and repent. This allows you to accept the responsibility and the consequences of your actions. This, of course, allows you to exit the spiral.

Secondly, if you don't confess and repent, you must find a way to shift the problem onto someone else. This is where the blame game begins. You will start blaming other people or their actions. You will focus on their faults instead of accepting responsibility. You may even start to ridicule, scorn, or use sarcasm to shift the blame. You essentially will do whatever it takes to get the spotlight off of yourself. Manipulation is a key that you always seem to have in your pocket.[86]

Blame also includes blaming yourself. Blaming yourself only gives the *illusion* that you're going to take responsibility. If you find yourself doing this, review Trigger #2—Shame. More than likely, you are dealing with a wounded shame story.

What's interesting here are the relational transitions that happen during the "blame game." You blame the very people you say you love. These are the people that mean the most to you. These are the people that you are willing to die for, yet you blame them for your behavior inside this trigger.

LOVING THE PLEASURE

We discussed the power of pleasure with temptation (Trigger #3) and hiddenness (Trigger #6). With blame, it comes up again, mainly because you haven't gotten real with God or yourself about the severity of your sin. You may say you want to change, but you are unwilling to do what is necessary for change itself. If you had, you wouldn't be playing the "blame game" at this moment. You might not admit it right now, but in some sick way, you still *love* the *pleasure* of your sin. In fact, you actually enjoy the *process* of the sex spiral—no matter how much you say you don't.

Keep in mind, talk is cheap at this point with your family. They are ready to see action. Playing the "blame game" keeps you in the spiral; and at some level, you enjoy the chaos, the chase, and the getaway. Its habit is livable. It doesn't really scare you anymore; and when it does, it tends to give you another adrenaline rush. What does scare you is living *without* pornography.

---

[86] England, Dorothy Marie. *Smoke & Mirrors: The Magical World of Chemical Dependency*. Cincinnati: Forward Movement, 1995.

Trigger #10: Blame

Eventually your fantasy world begins to seep into your real life when you refuse to exit the spiral by praying, fleeing, and confessing. When this happens, you unknowingly begin confusing reality with fantasy. This is where life really begins to hurt.

A LESSON FROM THE TV SHOW "FRIENDS"

In an episode of the television show "Friends," Chandler and Joey are flipping through the channels and accidentally come upon free porn. They are so excited about their discovery that they don't want to change the channel or turn off the television for fear of losing their new "gift" from the cable company. After what seems to be several days of watching nothing but pornography, Chandler comes in the front door and says to Joey, "I was just at the bank, and there was this really hot teller, and she didn't ask me to go 'do it' with her in the vault!"

Joey exclaims, "The same kind of thing happened to me! A woman-pizza-delivery-guy comes over, gives me the pizza, takes the money, and leaves!"

Chandler responds, "What? No 'nice apartment, I bet the bedrooms are huge?'"

Joey says, "No, nothing!"

Chandler responds, "Ya know what? We have to turn off the porn."

Joey replies, "I think you're right."

Chandler takes the remote and turns it off. Both Joey and Chandler wait for a moment in silence, and Joey says, "That's kind of nice."

"Yeah, that's kind of a relief," Chandler responds.

They wait for a few more moments, and then Chandler asks Joey, "Do you want to see if we still have it?"

Chandler clicks the remote, and the porn reappears. The closing scene is them celebrating.[87]

---

87 *Friends*. "The One with the Free Porn." Season 4, Episode 17. Directed by Michael Lembeck. Written by Richard Goodman. National Broadcasting Company, March 26, 1998.

This episode is funny. It's clever. However, behind the laughs is a dark, subtle truth. Pornography changes the way we think about people. We confuse real-life reality with perverse fantasy. We literally teach our brains how to sexualize everything and everyone; but when things don't go our way, we can bank on the fact that we will blame others throughout this process. Did you notice how Chandler and Joey both blamed the teller and the "woman-pizza-delivery-guy" for not wanting to have sex with them? Oh, the nerve!

WHO SAID YOU WERE NAKED?

Let's now transition from a situational comedy back to reality. In the historical account of the fall, Adam and Eve eat from the tree they were supposed to avoid and are now trying to hide somewhere in the garden. *"'Who told you that you were naked?' the Lord God asked. 'Have you eaten from the tree whose fruit I commanded you not to eat?' The man replied, 'It was the woman you gave me who gave me the fruit, and I ate it'"* (Gen. 3:11-12).

God asked Adam a yes-or-no question. Pretty straightforward, correct? Look what happens. Adam responds, "If You hadn't given me the woman, this wouldn't have happened." Do you see the implication here? Adam not only blames Eve, but he also has the audacity to blame God for creating the woman.

Genesis 3:13 shows us the woman's response: *"Then the Lord God asked the woman, 'What have you done?' 'The serpent deceived me,' she replied. 'That's why I ate it.'"* While Adam blamed both the woman and God, Eve places the blame on the serpent. Although she didn't take responsibility for her sin, she did expose Satan as a tempter and liar. Regardless, blame continues to plague us in our relationships today, especially when it comes to habitual sin like lust.

Trigger #10: Blame

WE'RE ALL GOING TO DIE!

Being blamed also does something to us on the receiving side of sin. If you are the spouse, you know this scenario all too well. Let's look at how blame impacted Moses one day while in the desert.

> *There was no water for the people to drink at that place, so they rebelled against Moses and Aaron. The people blamed Moses and said, "If only we had died in the Lord's presence with our brothers! Why have <u>you</u> brought the congregation of the Lord's people into this wilderness to die, along with all our livestock? Why did <u>you</u> make us leave Egypt and bring us here to this terrible place? This land has no grain, no figs, no grapes, no pomegranates, and no water to drink!" Moses and Aaron turned away from the people and went to the entrance of the Tabernacle, where they fell face down on the ground. Then the glorious presence of the Lord appeared to them, And the Lord said to Moses, "You and Aaron must take the staff and assemble the entire community. As the people watch, speak to the rock over there, and it will pour out its water. You will provide enough water from the rock to satisfy the whole community and their livestock."*
>
> *So Moses did as he was told. He took the staff from the place where it was kept before the Lord. Then he and Aaron summoned the people to come and gather at the rock. "Listen, you rebels!" he shouted. "Must we bring you water from this rock?" Then Moses raised his hand and struck the rock twice with the staff, and water gushed out. So the entire community and their livestock drank their fill. But the Lord said to Moses and Aaron, "Because you did not trust me enough to demonstrate my holiness to the people of Israel, you will not lead them into the land I am giving them!"* (Num. 20:2-12).

We see Moses dealing with anger throughout his life. As a young man, he killed an Egyptian (Exod. 2:12). Years later, he broke the first set of the Ten Commandments (Exod. 32:19). During this particular event, however, the Israelites blamed Moses for not having water. Moses responded by doing what he had done in the past—he sought the counsel of the Lord. The problem, however, is that Moses' heart wasn't right. He went before the Lord, but he did so while still frustrated and angry.

We see this by the way he spoke to the Israelites. His anger continued with his actions. Moses didn't follow the Lord's instructions exactly as stated. He became passive-aggressive and, in anger, did what he had previously done to the rock at Horeb (Exod. 17:6). He was told to *speak* to the rock, not strike it. It's important to understand that God did not punish Moses for simply not obeying Him; He punished Moses because he used God's power to perform a miracle that was previously done—only this time with anger. His anger prevented him from trusting God in a new way; therefore, God's holiness was not displayed. It certainly would have been an amazing miracle for everyone to witness Moses simply *speaking* to the rock to provide water, rather than using force. Astonishingly, God still allows the miracle to happen, even though Moses disobeyed.

This lesson is very important for friends and spouses walking with someone who is enslaved to pornography. This happened because Moses was the *recipient* of blame. He was the victim of other people's sin. We as humans don't know how to deal with this. When someone sins against us, we want to get even. Think of these opportunities as building your own spiritual muscle as you continue to grow in your own personal walk with the Lord.

Blaming others or being blamed keeps you in the spiral. To exit, you must repent. Repenting of the *process* of sin looks like this:
- Admit that you enjoy being in the spiral—from first being triggered to planning on how to hide, lie, and manipulate people so that you can commit the sin. Confess that you love your sin and truly enjoy engaging in the pleasure that it brings.

Trigger #10: Blame

- Realize that you actually have to give yourself permission to sin.
- Admit that your life plan (or lack thereof) is what got you where you currently are.
- Radically submit to another life plan—the biblical plan.
- Actually work God's plan for your life.

Not only does blame keep us in the spiral but it also launches us into the next trigger—anger.

CHAPTER 13

TRIGGER #11: ANGER

IN 1977, BURT REYNOLDS STARRED in a box office hit titled *Smokey and the Bandit*. He drove a black Pontiac Trans Am with T-Tops in the film. I'll never forget that car. My dad bought one just like it. I would sit in the passenger seat, and my younger brother would sit on the armrest while he drove. There weren't any seatbelt laws back then. Needless to say, safety was not much of a concern for my dad. Besides, what could possibly go wrong?

One weekend, I remember going through the car wash. Dad decided that instead of towel drying the car (like a normal person), he would simply drive really, *really*, fast to "air dry" it. I looked at the speedometer, and we were going over 100 mph through the suburban streets of Ft. Wayne, Indiana. I'm guessing the speed limit was 40 or 50 mph max.

After passing several cars at what seemed to be mach speed, dad finally had to slow down because of traffic. Some of the cars that we passed started catching up with us. One of the drivers that passed us gave us a certain hand gesture as he drove by. This gesture sent my dad into overdrive himself. He didn't say anything but decided to switch lanes very quickly as we pulled up to the red light. Dad tapped this car with his front bumper and then slammed on the gas pedal. The next thing I knew, his *Smokey and the Bandit* Pontiac Trans Am was screeching and spinning its tires while grey smoke filled up the intersection! I specifically remember the passenger looking back at us in terror. After a few seconds, dad started pushing this car out into the middle of the intersection with oncoming traffic. The driver finally released his own brake, slammed on the gas, ran the red light, and drove off into safety.

"Dad, why'd you do that?" I asked.

"Because he gave your dad 'the bird,'" he responded in defiance.

"What's 'the bird'?" I asked.

My dad showed me this hand gesture (the middle finger) that I've never seen before. "This is 'the bird,' son, and *no one* gives it to your dad."

THE REAL REASON

When people go for counseling, they usually say that pornography is the biggest problem in their lives. Porn is not the *real* reason they go for help. It's a symptom to a much deeper issue. The real problem is the same problem we all have—a strained relationship with Jesus Christ.

The reason my dad lost his mind on the road that day isn't because a stranger gave him an obscene hand gesture. It was because my dad didn't have any peace in his life. He was an alcoholic and a sex addict. These things that he used to medicate his pain actually made him a very angry man because that's what habitual sin does in our lives. Whenever we attach ourselves to a cheap substitute, an underlying and constant frustration settles in. This is fertile ground for strongholds to take root as well. When we break God's moral laws and continue to live outside of God's will for our lives, we become angry. We become angry because it's impossible to find peace apart from the blood-stained cross of Jesus Christ, who is the Prince of Peace (Isa. 9:6).

Unfortunately, my dad and I never really got along. I loved him, but I never really understood him. I never figured out why he constantly had a beer in one hand and women on his mind until it was too late. Truth be told, I judged my dad for drinking. I didn't like it. It seemed that whenever my brother and I stayed with dad, we spent a lot of time at the local bar. My dad was like "Norm" from the TV show "Cheers." Everyone at the bar knew him and loved him. He was accepted. That bar was dad's community.

It's one thing to be addicted to pornography. It's quite another to drink on top of it. Dad was *comorbid*. He dealt with two addictions at the same time—alcohol and pornography. The term really kind of says it all, doesn't it? Co-*morbid*. When we speak on habitual sin and addiction, it's important to know that alcohol is a gateway drug to pornography. It's very easy to let our guard down (a.k.a. morality and conscience) to have a few beers and then start looking at pornography.

ANGER

Trigger #11 is Anger. Pornography and anger are two sides of the same coin. You can't have one without the other. In other words, you can't view pornography over time and *not* be angry.

I found this to be unbelievably true in my own life. I was constantly angry. My life seemed to simmer with frustration. When something or someone would bump into me, my anger would spew out like lava from a volcano. I never really understood the source of that frustration until I recognized the power that the sin of pornography had over my life.

> **When you follow the desires of your sinful nature, the results are very clear: sexual immorality, impurity, lustful pleasures, idolatry, sorcery, hostility, quarreling, jealousy, outbursts of anger, selfish ambition, dissension, division, envy, drunkenness, wild parties, and other sins like these. Let me tell you again, as I have before, that anyone living that sort of life will not inherit the Kingdom of God** (Gal. 5:19-21).

Pornography and anger are two sides of same coin for a very specific reason. I believe it's one of God's natural laws—a moral principle deemed for all human behavior. In other words, when you choose to look at porn, you unknowingly choose to be angry.

Stay with me. God created mankind in His own image. As we discussed in "Chapter 1: Biblical Sexuality," when both husband and wife come together in a sexual union, God is honored and glorified. Needless to say, He does not blush. However, when we watch pornography, we are stepping outside of God's will for our lives and breaking His moral law. We are watching something that is holy and sacred between a man and his wife. Pornography takes this holy union and desecrates it. Remember our definition of pornography? It's the "emotional, spiritual, and physical abuse of people performing profane acts of sexuality for the arousal of a viewer or audience."

Sexuality is sacred. When you strip the holiness out of it, something begins to happen to your being. It's your spirit telling you that an injustice has taken place—the injustice of watching something that is supposed to be experienced (not watched) only under a covenant relationship with God between husband and wife. Pornography makes you angry because you're a third party. You are viewing an act, although holy and sacred, that is now scarred with sin because of your presence.

GOD AND ANGER

Biblical counselor and founder of *Hope for Your Heart*, June Hunt, teaches there are four common sources of anger: hurt, injustice, fear, and frustration.[88] There are also two types of anger—righteous and unrighteous anger.

Our culture loves to think of baby Jesus or the meek, mild, sissified Jesus. Thankfully, this interpretation is not from the counsel of God. For example, did you know that God gets angry? Psalm 7:11 reads, **"God is an honest judge. He is angry with the wicked every day."**

Did you know that believers are *commanded* to be angry? The apostle Paul writes in Ephesians 4:26 (ESV), **"Be angry and do not sin; do not let the sun go down on your anger."**[89] What are we commanded to be angry over? When we review the four common sources of anger, injustice stands out from the other three. Hurt, fear, and frustration are about self. Injustice, on the other hand, is about others. We are

---
88 Hunt, June. *Anger: Facing the Fire Within*. Self-Published, 2011.
89 *The Holy Bible: English Standard Version*. Wheaton: Standard Bible Society, 2016.

commanded by God to get angry when we see injustice happening to another person.

Let's look at a couple of examples of when Jesus got angry.

> *Again he entered the synagogue, and a man was there with a withered hand. And they watched Jesus, to see whether he would heal him on the Sabbath, so that they might accuse him. And he said to the man with the withered hand, "Come here." And he said to them, "Is it lawful on the Sabbath to do good or to do harm, to save life or to kill?" But they were silent. And he looked around at them with anger, grieved at their hardness of heart, and said to the man, "Stretch out your hand." He stretched it out, and his hand was restored. The Pharisees went out and immediately held counsel with the Herodians against him, how to destroy him* (Mk. 3:1-6—ESV).[90]

Why was Jesus angry? Was it because the Pharisees were trying to kill Him? No, but wouldn't you at least be a little upset if people were trying to kill you? Of course, you would, but not Jesus. Jesus was angry because of the injustice toward this man with the crippled hand. The pastors, priests, and ministers of that day *prevented* people from getting well. They made it intentionally hard to find God and have a relationship with Him. They preferred law instead of grace because the law was all about their own career and performance. It was about doing certain things a specific way. This kept them pure—or so they thought. Their *working* at holiness put the spotlight on them instead of God. That's why they despised Jesus and His grace. Jesus was offering a gift that they were unwilling to accept.

> *It was nearly time for the Jewish Passover celebration, so Jesus went to Jerusalem. In the Temple area he saw merchants selling cattle, sheep, and doves for sacrifices; he also saw dealers at tables exchanging foreign money. Jesus made a whip from some ropes and chased them all out of the Temple. He*

---

90 Ibid.

drove out the sheep and cattle, scattered the money changers' coins over the floor, and turned over their tables. Then, going over to the people who sold doves, he told them, "Get these things out of here. Stop turning my Father's house into a marketplace!" Then his disciples remembered this prophecy from the scriptures: "Passion for God's house will consume me (Jn. 2:13-17).

Why was Jesus angry this time? The Jews turned the temple into a shopping mall! They defiled the temple, which represented the presence of God Himself. The celebration of the Passover turned into a way to make a quick buck. The main desire and intention of the crowd was greed, instead of worshipping God.

Notice that these examples of Jesus becoming angry didn't have anything to do with Jesus Himself, but were rather a holy defense for God and others. Jesus was angry because of the injustice that was happening toward people. This is called righteous anger.

THE THREE TYPES OF PORNIFIED ANGER

Why do you and I get angry? It's usually not out of concern for others. We get angry because of the following reasons:

It's the fastest way to control the situation. If you rise up and raise your voice or become aggressive in some way, you're trying to make everyone else submit to your authority. It's an illusion of control in your own mind, but it proves how out of control you are to others. Anger is also a result of:

- You're not getting your way.
- You're not being treated the way you think you should be treated.
- You've been disrespected and/or humiliated.
- Someone or something is in your way. They are blocking a goal or expectation.

- Your expectations of life, work, family, children, and money are all too high.

Now let's consider what kind of anger arises when you get caught looking at pornography. Review the four common sources of anger—hurt, injustice, fear, and frustration—and think about which type of anger you feel. For example:

1. I'm now *hurt*—I'm embarrassed (unrighteous anger).
2. I'm *fearful* of the future, the consequences, and what others think of me (unrighteous anger).
3. I'm *frustrated* that no one understands me, and I'm frustrated with myself because I'm unwilling to ask for real help (unrighteous anger).

Above, I have three out of the four sources of anger listed. Notice that those three all have to do with self. They are all *unrighteous*. Injustice (righteous anger) is the only one not listed, and that is because it has to do with other people. Anger is usually about "me, myself, and I," which is the unholy trinity.[91] And when your anger is about this "trinity," you'll use anger to try and control the situation.

- James 4:1-3—**"What is causing the quarrels and fights among you? Don't they come from the evil desires at war within you? You want what you don't have, so you scheme and kill to get it. You are jealous of what others have, but you can't get it, so you fight and wage war to take it away from them. Yet you don't have what you want because you don't ask God for it. And even when you ask, you don't get it because your motives are all wrong—you want only what will give you <u>pleasure</u> (emphasis mine)."**
- Proverbs 14:17—**"Short-tempered people do foolish things, and schemers are hated."**

---

91 DelHousaye, Darryl. "The President's Class." Class lecture, Scottsdale Bible Church, Scottsdale, AZ, 2009.

- Proverbs 22:24-25—*"**Don't befriend angry people or associate with hot-tempered people, or you will learn to be like them and endanger your soul.**"*
- Proverbs 29:11—*"**Fools vent their anger, but the wise quietly hold it back.**"*
- James 1:20—*"**Human anger does not produce the righteousness God desires.**"*

UNRESOLVED ANGER

Lastly, we must address *unresolved* anger. Do you know the exact reason *why* you become angry? Starting with the four sources of anger is a huge step in the right direction. But let me ask it another way—do you know why you are grumpy, grouchy, irritable, or short-tempered a lot of the time? Would people use words like these to describe you? If so, there is a good possibility that you are living with unresolved anger.

It's one thing to be angry over a situation or event. It's another thing entirely to not know why you have a chronic sense of frustration in your life. Unresolved anger is dangerous because there hasn't been a solution to a problem in your past. Without a solution, your past controls your future. So many of us make critical life-altering decisions from our shame story discussed in chapter four. But the apostle Paul writes in Philippians 3:13b-14, *"**I focus on this one thing: Forgetting the past and looking forward to what lies ahead, I press on to reach the end of the race and receive the heavenly prize for which God, through Christ Jesus, is calling us.**"*

For us to forget the past, we must address the past. It's been said that we must relive to forgive. There is a biblical way to address these issues—a system and process to once and for all address the hurt, shame, and trauma that have plagued us for years and even decades. I would encourage you to seek out a trusted biblical counselor to start.

But what happens when you refuse to ask for help and continue to live with unresolved anger? Well, you end up doing really stupid

Trigger #11: ANGER

things like using your *Smokey and the Bandit* Pontiac Trans Am to push another car through the intersection with your children in the car.

If we choose to not exit the spiral sooner or later, we will reach Trigger #12—Hopelessness.

CHAPTER 14

TRIGGER #12: HOPELESSNESS

I KNOW WHERE THE GUN is. This thought leaped from my mind as I woke up from a nap one day. I was supposed to be working, but my depression was so bad that I physically couldn't stay awake. Yes, I knew exactly where the gun was. It was just down the street at a pawn shop, along with my second wife's wedding ring and some other things we had to pawn just to keep food on the table.

My life sucked. I divorced my first wife and left her for another woman (on whom I was already cheating). I also couldn't keep a job to save my life. I was fired from a job every other month—a total of nine jobs in less than eighteen months. My depression was unbearable. It was too heavy, and I didn't want to stay awake. For a year and a half, all I wanted to do was sleep. On top of all that drama, I couldn't stand this woman that I had been completely obsessed with and was now married to. I was finding out that two decades of living in sexual sin makes a person very, *very* stupid.

That was the day that I decided to kill myself. I understood that I was the end result of my decisions. I realized (once again) how much of a loser I was. I saw how many people I had hurt and was still hurting. I saw that I was unable to take care of myself, let alone a new wife and her teenage son. I had no hope. *All is lost. Nothing will ever change. I'm a freak and a pervert. Why not kill myself? WHY NOT?* I raged. After all, I've only been thinking about it for the past year, and no one will miss me.

The apostle Paul tells us that **"the wages of sin is death"** (Rom. 6:23a). At that moment in my life, it was very apparent that I was receiving all of those wages at one time. I was reaping what I had planted—a life full of drama and pain. I fooled myself into thinking that my life would be different somehow. I truly thought that I could live my life *my way* and that God would somehow ignore it and even bless it at times. After all, boys will be boys. Well, I was wrong. Dead wrong.

As soon as the thought to kill myself went through my head, I heard this question, *That's great. So, you're going to carry on the family tradition of being a coward? Your grandfather shot himself; your father drank himself to death; and now it's your turn?* I thought about that question (oblivious to Who even asked it) and got up and went back to work that day. I wish I could say that was the day that I made the decision to exit the spiral. It wasn't. I spent the next couple of years continuing to spiral through it. Some days hurt so bad, I would just binge up to a half a dozen times per day. God, in essence, said, "You want this, so here ya go. I'm going to allow you so much sex, you'll vomit from it." The apostle Paul writes in Romans 1:24-29:

> **So God abandoned them to do whatever shameful things their hearts desired. As a result, they did vile and degrading things with each other's bodies. They traded the truth about God for a lie. So they worshiped and served the things God created instead of the Creator himself, who is worthy of eternal praise! Amen. That is why God abandoned them to their shameful desires. Even the women turned against the natural way to have sex and instead indulged in sex with each other. And the men, instead of having normal sexual relations with women, burned with lust for each other. Men did shameful things with other men, and as a result of this sin, they suffered within themselves the penalty they deserved. Since they thought it foolish to acknowledge God, he abandoned them to their foolish thinking and let them do things that should never be done. Their lives became full of every kind of wickedness, sin, greed, hate, envy, murder, quarreling, deception, malicious behavior, and gossip.**

God did, indeed, allow me to indulge in shameful desires. I did whatever I wanted, and my life was a complete train wreck because of it. God had delivered on His promises—as He always does. He gave me up to my lust. He gave me up to my dishonorable passions and debased mind.

HOPELESSNESS

The last trigger in *The Sex Spiral* is hopelessness. There is nothing worse than thinking that my life would *never* change. This is why I considered suicide. Even in the diary of my darkest days, I yearned for just a glimpse of hope. I never really wanted to die; I just wanted the pain to go away. I hoped in hope, but at the end of the day, I was unwilling to change. I was unwilling to stop looking at pornography.

I learned that guilt and shame don't go away on their own. Not resolving these issues in your life will lead to the loss of hope. Over time, you will also lose your motivation to even try.

The choice to not trust God and others with your sin leads to bondage. When you don't learn to trust in what Jesus did on the cross, you will continue to remain in bondage to the sex spiral.

THE LAW OF DIMINISHING RETURNS

The law of diminishing returns (through this lens of lust) dictates that you can never go back to the simple, innocent days of what first gave you pleasure. The more you look at porn, the more porn you need. So, porn is not just a liar, but a thief as well. It's a thief because it not only steals your innocence but also your time. What was attractive at the beginning is no longer stimulating. That's why you are not a slave to just one image. You need *more* stimuli, which are the graphic images. Eventually, the porn becomes so disgusting and dehumanizing, you realize that the materials you are looking at are beyond belief. At the same time, you have a hard time asking for help because of the shame involved. Before you know it, twenty years fly by and you'll ask, *How did I get to the place in my life where I'm hiding in a closet with a loaded gun acting like a coward?*

Hopelessness launches us past Trigger #1 (Awareness) right into Trigger #2 (Shame). Keep in mind that you don't start where you left off. This is not a cycle, but a spiral. It's not linear; it's messy; it deepens ever so subtly. Over time, your pornography use becomes more perverse and demonic. Eventually, pornography won't be enough for you to get your fix. You'll need to move to the real thing.

I mentioned in the introduction that one of my goals in writing this book was to answer the question posed by the apostle Paul in Romans 7:24b: *"Who will free me from this life that is dominated by sin and death?"* Are you ready for the answer? Good. Before we get there, however, let's get some encouragement from a surprising source.

CHAPTER 15

THE ANSWER: LIVING IN FREEDOM

HAVE YOU EVER WATCHED THE opening ceremony of the Olympics? It's quite the production, isn't it? A tremendous amount of ceremonial pomp and splendor, mixed with music, video, lights, and performers. Why not? After all, these athletes have been training most of their lives for this opportunity to compete. Three hundred events in thirty-five different sports over sixteen days. And then it's over. The lights get turned off; the spectators go home; and it's back to training. Four more years of grinding it out day after day, all for the opportunity of temporary athletic glory.

Think of the early mornings these athletes get up to train, resisting the urge to hit snooze and roll over in bed—rain or shine, snow or sleet. These athletes have given up a lot of things like junk food, entertainment, and even certain relationships to be the best of the very best. They sacrifice and push their bodies through the emotional, spiritual, and physical pain in order to achieve victory. Why? Each athlete certainly has their own reason, but you can bank on the fact that they don't picture themselves taking second place. They picture themselves at the grand opening ceremony. They have visions of receiving the gold medal around their neck, waving to the crowd, and singing their national anthem in celebration.

It's a dream of a lifetime to compete, let alone win a medal. The Olympics represent the ultimate in competition for amateur athletes. Thousands of athletes traveling from the four corners of the world participate. When you arrive here, there is no more training and no more preparation. It's "go time." Can you imagine that feeling as a competitor?

It's inspiring to see people push themselves to the very limits of athletic perfection. This is why we watch; this is why we cheer. The Olympics remind me of the old television show called, "The Wide World of Sports." The voiceover to the show said, "The thrill of victory and the agony of defeat! The human drama of athletic competition." Isn't that what the Olympics really are—a human drama featuring athletic competition?

COME DREAM WITH ME

I want you to picture *yourself* as one of those athletes. Yes, *you* are walking into a stadium filled with tens of thousands of cheering people. *You* are walking in the Parade of Nations, watching firsthand the hanging of the Olympic flag, singing the Olympic anthem, taking the Olympic oath, and watching the Olympic flame being lit. However, as you look around at the spectators in the stadium, you start to notice something unusual. Wait, these people aren't mere spectators; they are spiritual athletes of the past![92] In fact, these are Hall of Faith members who have run and finished the same race that you are now competing in (Heb. 11).

You see our forefathers—Abraham, Isaac, and Jacob—all holding huge signs with *your* name! You see Moses and Joshua with their fists pumping in the air chanting, "Strong and Courageous! Strong and Courageous! Strong and Courageous" (Josh. 1:6, 7, 9, 18).

You look up in the box seats and see King David and King Solomon standing and clapping their hands in honor of *you*. The minor prophets are with them—Joel, Jonah, and Malachi all doing "the wave"! Isaiah, Jeremiah, and Daniel (the major prophets) are just a section below them, giving you the thumbs up.

---

92 Hughs, R. Kent. *Hebrews: An Anchor for the Soul*. Wheaton: Crossway Publishers, 2015.

The Answer: Living in Freedom

You look across the stadium, and you see Peter, James, and John, along with the rest of the apostles, giving each other "high-fives." Just when you think you've seen it all, you see the apostle Paul with Timothy, looking directly at *you* giving *you* a standing ovation! You can hardly believe your eyes! And lastly, you start to see your friends and family who have passed away—gone to be with the Lord—sitting in the front row, cheering *you* on as well.

They have all finished *their* own race. They continued running when there was *no* tangible evidence of seeing or knowing the outcome. They all struggled and chose temporary hardships for eternal honor.[93] All of them doubted and feared, and many of them wanted to quit—just like us. But their faith was demonstrated (not just talked about) through endurance, discipline, and suffering.

This imagery, my friend, is our motivation to never, ever give up. The motivation to learn and experience what it means to be forgiven and free from pornography is found in Hebrews 12:1-2 (ESV).[94] Let's break down this verse in sections to grasp it completely. There are ten sections total. I've written the Scripture verses out and have bolded the section that will be our focus. My suggestion is to read these verses out loud, emphasizing the text that is bolded, as you finish this chapter. This will allow you to start memorizing these two verses. I would also suggest stopping here and taking a few minutes to pray and ask the Holy Spirit to reveal new things to you as you read.

1. "Therefore, since we are surrounded by so great a cloud of witnesses . . ."

> **Therefore, since we are surrounded by so great a cloud of witnesses,** *let us also lay aside every weight, and sin which clings so closely, and let us run with endurance the race that is set before us, looking to Jesus, the founder and perfecter of our faith, who for the joy that was set before him endured the cross, despising the shame, and is seated at the right hand of the throne of God* (Heb. 12:1-2).

---

93 DeSilva, D. A. *Perseverance in Gratitude: A Socio-rhetorical Commentary on the Epistle "to the Hebrews."* Grand Rapids: Wm. B. Eerdmans Publishing Co., 2000. 436.
94 *The Holy Bible: English Standard Version.* Wheaton: Standard Bible Society, 2016.

Hebrews 11 is known as the Hall of Faith. It lists people in the Old Testament who lived their lives with faith in God—not perfect faith but persistent faith. This is why Hebrews 12:1 starts with "therefore." The author is pointing us back to the people listed in the previous chapter. These people are metaphorically "a cloud of witnesses" that have gone before us and are proof that we can finish this race and finish well—just like they did! These witnesses are not just passive spectators or armchair quarterbacks. No, no, no. These are people who know *exactly* what it's like to run this race called the Christian life.

2. "Let us also lay aside every weight . . ."

> *Therefore, since we are surrounded by so great a cloud of witnesses,* **let us also lay aside every weight,** *and sin which clings so closely, and let us run with endurance the race that is set before us, looking to Jesus, the founder and perfecter of our faith, who for the joy that was set before him endured the cross, despising the shame, and is seated at the right hand of the throne of God.*

"Laying aside every weight" means that we must strip ourselves of anything and everything that will hinder our performance. From a practical standpoint, we wouldn't run a marathon wearing hiking boots and a long, flowing boxing robe, would we? Those items are for other sports. If you watch the Olympics, you've obviously noticed that the contestants run with as little clothing as possible. This obviously can be quite the struggle for those of us who deal with lust. Even the Greeks who started the games ran practically naked.

From a spiritual standpoint, you must *learn* to run *light*. There is much to be said about living a simple, light life. You must lay aside any worldly hindrance, burden, stumbling block, or potential embarrassments to your Christ-centered faith.[95] Things like ambition, anger, fame, fear, and unforgiveness are all heavy. Each item carries its own

---

95 Vincent, M. R. *Word Studies in the New Testament.* Vol. 4. New York: Charles Scribner's Sons, 1887. 537.

weight—especially things from your past that have not been dealt with like emotional, physical, and sexual abuse and trauma. Even the things that you may consider as innocent must go if they are going to slow you down. All that does not help, hinders. It is by running that he learns what these things are. So long as he stands, he does not feel that they are burdensome and hampering.[96] Isn't that interesting? It's only when you start to run the race that you start to feel the full baggage of your life.

3. "And sin which clings so closely . . ."

> *Therefore, since we are surrounded by so great a cloud of witnesses, let us also lay aside every weight,* **and sin which clings so closely***, and let us run with endurance the race that is set before us, looking to Jesus, the founder and perfecter of our faith, who for the joy that was set before him endured the cross, despising the shame, and is seated at the right hand of the throne of God.*

The habitual sin of the Hebrews was unbelief. For you and me, it's lust (combined with the unbelief that we will never be truly free). Our lust keeps us from truly believing that life can actually change for good. It's the sin that continues to entangle, grip, and squeeze. It certainly does "cling so closely," doesn't it? It doesn't ever seem to let up or let go. There seems to be a test or temptation at every corner. For us to run this race, lust *must* be cast aside.

4. "And let us run with endurance the race that is set before us . . ."

> *Therefore, since we are surrounded by so great a cloud of witnesses, let us also lay aside every weight, and sin which clings so closely,* **and let us run with endurance the race that is set before us,** *looking to Jesus, the founder and perfecter of our faith, who*

---

[96] Gaebelein, Frank E., *The Expositor's Bible Commentary, Volume 12: Hebrews through Revelation.* Nashville: Zondervan, 1982.

for the joy that was set before him endured the cross, despising the shame, and is seated at the right hand of the throne of God.

We must *run*. We must *move*. It's every Christian's responsibility. We can't stay parked and *just* pray for our lust to miraculously go away. Let me give you an example. Over the past several years, I've been thinking a lot about exercise. Praying and thinking about exercise doesn't do much good, does it? It's only when I get my body moving and discipline myself to not stuff my face with bacon double cheeseburgers that I actually start losing weight. It does not matter how much I pray to lose weight. God will never honor that prayer if I'm unwilling to learn discipline and self-control.

The same principle applies to breaking free from pornography. You must pray *and* run this race. The Christian life is not a sprint. Your goal is to run the race that God has given *you*—not to run someone else's. When you persevere to the end, it's God who will declare you a winner. This is a life-changing, life-altering, long-distance race that requires *imperfect* perseverance and elasticity. Understanding forgiveness and becoming free from pornography takes patience, persistence, and tenacity. It's starting small and walking slow. It's about implementing a plan (the one you have in your hands) soaked in prayer and letting nothing—and God means nothing—get in your way of finishing well.

The Greek word for "race" in this verse is *agōn*. It literally means "a contest, conflict or struggle."[97] We get our word *agony* from it. *Agony* is this idea of "extreme physical or mental suffering." It's prolonged pain.

It is believed that Greece is the birthplace of the Olympics. Some athletes back then participated in a *pentathlon*—a contest featuring five events:
1. Long Jump
2. Javelin Throw
3. Discus Throw

---

97 Schwandt, John. *The English Greek Reverse Interlinear New Testament English Standard Version.* Lexham Press, 2009.

4. Foot race
5. Wrestling

All five events were performed *on the same day*. Now can you imagine doing all these events and then wrestling someone at the very end? *Agony!* It's speaking of having a grueling fight until you have nothing left to give. The fight has taken everything out of you. You have essentially left everything out on the field.[98] The Greeks found this style of training beneficial as it prepared these athletes for war. *This* is why the writer uses the word *agony*.

My last thought on this section is that if *we* are running an agonizing race, that means there must be competitors, right? I would say we have a definite group of opponents—the world, our flesh, and Satan (Eph. 2:1-3)—who want to steal, kill, and destroy everything in our lives (Jn. 10:10). The problem with our opponents is that we can't see them. Satan wants to steal your time, so you can be unproductive for the Kingdom of God. He wants to kill all your godly relationships, so you stay isolated and alone. And he wants to destroy your marriage, so you can lose your witness for Christ.

5. "Looking to Jesus, the founder and perfecter of our faith . . ."

> *Therefore, since we are surrounded by so great a cloud of witnesses, let us also lay aside every weight, and sin which clings so closely, and let us run with endurance the race that is set before us,* **looking to Jesus, the founder and perfecter of our faith,** *who for the joy that was set before him endured the cross, despising the shame, and is seated at the right hand of the throne of God.*

We are to constantly look to Jesus as we run. We are to get our eyes off our sin and onto our Savior. If we don't, we will fail (Matt. 14:22-33).

---

98 Ford, Nick. *Suffering & Endurance*, May 22, 2016. http://nhcc-az.com/sermons/hebrews/mediaposts/suffering-and-endurance.

We are not to look to the Hall of Faith members in the stands or to Mohammed, Buddha, or Joseph Smith, but to *Jesus*. Jesus is the *only One* who came from heaven to run this agonizing race and to give us a perfect example of what faith in His Father looked like (Jn. 3:13, 6:38).

I love how the author of Hebrews focuses on the human side of our Savior. We are to look to *Jesus*—not the Christ (the Messiah), but to *Jesus*. Jesus Christ was fully human and fully God. It's called the *hypostatic union* (if you want to use a big, swanky, theological term); but at the end of the day, God's humanity and divinity are a mystery. By looking to *Jesus*, the author points us to a very personal, human relationship with our Lord. It's on a first-name basis.

From a practical level, what happens when a hurdle jumper becomes distracted by looking at the people in the stands? Would they start slowing down? Miss a hurdle? You bet. And the moment we take our eyes off Jesus, the same thing happens to us spiritually.

"The Founder and Perfecter of our faith" could also be translated as *Pioneer*. This is the only place in the New Testament that this particular Greek word is used.[99] By definition, a pioneer is someone who is the first to do something. Jesus not only pioneered fulfilling every single Old Testament law, but He also blazed a new trail called *grace*. Jesus didn't just pioneer your freedom from pornography, but He also perfected it through His death and resurrection.

6. "Who for the joy . . ."

> *Therefore, since we are surrounded by so great a cloud of witnesses, let us also lay aside every weight, and sin which clings so closely, and let us run with endurance the race that is set before us, looking to Jesus, the founder and perfecter of our faith,* **who for the joy** *that was set before him endured the cross, despising the shame, and is seated at the right hand of the throne of God.*

---

99 Allen, D. L. *Hebrews*. Nashville: B & H Publishing Group, 2010. 574.

The Answer: Living in Freedom

This *joy* is a joy that Jesus would later have after His work was done. It's delayed gratification. It's the same joy that He had with His Father before They created the world and everything in it. Jesus speaks of this joy in John 17:4-5, ***"I brought glory to you here on earth by completing the work you gave me to do. Now, Father, bring me into the glory we shared before the world began."*** Jesus is speaking of that joy when He personally exchanged our (sexual) guilt and shame for His death and resurrection.

7. "That was set before him . . ."

> *Therefore, since we are surrounded by so great a cloud of witnesses, let us also lay aside every weight, and sin which clings so closely, and let us run with endurance the race that is set before us, looking to Jesus, the founder and perfecter of our faith, who for the joy* **that was set before him** *endured the cross, despising the shame, and is seated at the right hand of the throne of God.*

Several years ago, Amy and I had ministry friends who sent us on a cruise. It was an incredible experience—just us and 4,000 of our closest friends. Amy and I could do anything we wanted to do. We saw several shows, ate when and where we wanted, went to the pool, read books, etc. They even had rock climbing and a surfing pool. Being on the cruise reminded me of how God's will works. There is His permissive will and His perfect will. God's *permissive* will allowed Amy and I to do whatever we wanted on the cruise. The one thing that we could not do is go tell the captain where our next destination should be. The course had already been precisely set by the captain. It was mapped out. This is an example of God's *perfect* will. From a spiritual perspective, God has a specific destination for us. He commands us to be holy and pure. The apostle Paul writes in 1 Thessalonians 4:3-4, **"God's will is for you to be holy, so stay away from all sexual sin. Then each of you will control his own body and live in holiness and honor."** Paul also writes in Ephesians 5:3 (NIV),

"But among you there must not be even a hint of sexual immorality, or of any kind of impurity, or of greed, because these are improper for God's holy people."[100]

8. "Endured the cross . . ."

> Therefore, since we are surrounded by so great a cloud of witnesses, let us also lay aside every weight, and sin which clings so closely, and let us run with endurance the race that is set before us, looking to Jesus, the founder and perfecter of our faith, who for the joy that was set before him **endured the cross,** despising the shame, and is seated at the right hand of the throne of God.

Jesus *endured* the cross for you. He suffered painfully and patiently. There is not a more painful way to die. The Romans were perfecters of pain. D.A. DeSilva writes:

> The form of execution called crucifixion was calculated to leave the victim utterly stripped of dignity and worth in the eyes of this world. It was the vilest, most degrading death possible, as the crucified was hung up before all the world precisely as an example of how not to act. A shameful death was the most feared of evils among many ancients since it left one with no opportunity to regain one's honor. The last word on one's life was a judgment of worthlessness.[101]

Jesus was *made* sin for you (2 Cor. 5:21). This means that your (sexual) sins were transferred to Him for the sole purpose of the Father's holy and righteous punishment.

---

100 *The Holy Bible: The New International Version.* Grand Rapids: Zondervan, 2011.
101 DeSilva, D. A. *Perseverance in Gratitude: A Socio-rhetorical Commentary on the Epistle "to the Hebrews."* Grand Rapids: Wm. B. Eerdmans Publishing Co., 2000.

9. "Despising the shame . . ."

Therefore, since we are surrounded by so great a cloud of witnesses, let us also lay aside every weight, and sin which clings so closely, and let us run with endurance the race that is set before us, looking to Jesus, the founder and perfecter of our faith, who for the joy that was set before him endured the cross, **despising the shame,** *and is seated at the right hand of the throne of God.*

In most (if not all) pictures that I have seen of the crucifixion, Jesus has some type of covering around His waist. However, Roman soldiers didn't care about modesty. Jesus was crucified completely naked. There was no clothing to protect our Lord from disgrace. Jesus was without a shred of decency or dignity as He struggled to breathe, hanging from the blood-stained, wooden cross. Look at the following Scripture:

- Matthew 27:35—**"After they had nailed him to the cross, the soldiers gambled for his clothes by throwing dice."**
- Mark 15:24—**"Then the soldiers nailed him to the cross. They divided his clothes and threw dice to decide who would get each piece."**
- Luke 23:34—**"Jesus said, 'Father, forgive them, for they don't know what they are doing.' And the soldiers gambled for his clothes by throwing dice."**
- John 19:23-24 (ESV)—**"When the soldiers had crucified Jesus, they took his garments and divided them into four parts, one part for each soldier; also his tunic. But the tunic was seamless, woven in one piece from top to bottom, so they said to one another, 'Let us not tear it, but cast lots for it to see whose it shall be.' This was to fulfill the scripture which says, 'They divided my garments among them, and for my clothing they cast lots.'"**

The tunic that these Roman soldiers gambled for was similar to our underwear. Jesus was *beyond* humiliation and embarrassment. J. Vernon McGee writes:

He was crucified naked. It is difficult for us in this age of nudity and pornography to comprehend the great humiliation He suffered by hanging nude on the cross. Despising the shame is the same concept as *despising public opinion*. Jesus disregarded and disdained the shame of the world. In saying that He "despised" shame, the author of Hebrews points out that Jesus understood public opinion to be based on error and ignorance. It is only the approval of God, Christ, and the community of faith across the ages that should determine their choices and actions.[102]

P.T. O'Brien says, "He 'despised the shame' and overturned the opinions and values of the world. They were not worthy of being taken into account when it was a question of His obedience to the will of God."[103] People thought that dying on a cross was a terrible disgrace, but Jesus didn't think so. It was as if Jesus took your sexual shame and just cast it off as if it were nothing. It held no value, which means that it now holds no power over you. The apostle John writes in 1 John 4:4, **"But you belong to God, my dear children. You have already won a victory over those people, because the Spirit who lives in you is greater than the spirit who lives in the world."** The apostle Paul writes in Romans 8:31, **"What shall we say about such wonderful things as these? If God is for us, who can ever be against us?"**

10. "And is seated at the right hand of the throne of God . . ."

Therefore, since we are surrounded by so great a cloud of witnesses, let us also lay aside every weight, and sin which clings so closely, and let us run with endurance the race that is set before us, looking to Jesus, the founder and perfecter of our faith, who for the joy that

---

102 Ibid.
103 Ellingworth, P., and E.A. Nida. *A Handbook on the Letter to the Hebrews.* New York: United Bible Societies, 1994. 291.

was set before him endured the cross, despising the shame, **and is seated at the right hand of the throne of God.**

Jesus *sat down.* His work is finished. He doesn't ever have to repeat what He did. The high priests in the Old Testament had to continue slaughtering lambs to make atonement for the people of Israel over and over. Jesus, on the other hand, *was* the Lamb of God who once and for all took away the (sexual) sin of the world (Jn. 1:29, 1:36, 1 Pet. 1:19).

Jesus now sits at the right hand of His Father—in all the glory and majesty from when time first began. It's a position of preeminence and supremacy. It's a place reserved only for the King of all kings—One who ultimately rules and reigns the entire universe.

THE UNANSWERED QUESTION

I have discovered this principle of life—that when I want to do what is right, I inevitably do what is wrong. I love God's law with all my heart. But there is another power within me that is at war with my mind. This power makes me a slave to the sin that is still within me. Oh, what a miserable person I am! Who will free me from this life that is dominated by sin and death? (Rom. 7:21-24).

What, other than death, can free him from a body that craves sin more powerfully than his mind craves righteousness?[104] It's the "old man" who rarely seems to go away. For you and me, it's the lustful bent we view the world through. Will this "old man" *ever* go away? Yes, but he doesn't go away without a fight, and, as my friend and colleague Mark Laaser says, "It's the 'fight of your life.'"[105]

I love how Paul answers his own question in the very next verse: **"Thank God! The answer is in Jesus Christ our Lord"** (Rom. 7:25a). Jesus

---

104 Swindoll, Chuck. *Insights on Romans.* Grand Rapids: Zondervan, 2010.
105 Clinton, Timothy and Dr. Mark Laaser. *The Fight of Your Life: Manning Up to the Challenge of Sexual Integrity.* Shippensburg: Destiny Image Publishers, Inc., 2015.

Christ is the *reason* we run! *He* is our prize! *He* is the finish line, and the Kingdom of God is our reward. Paul also writes in 1 Corinthians 9:24-27:

> **Don't you realize that in a race everyone runs, but only one person gets the prize? So run to win! All athletes are disciplined in their training. They do it to win a prize that will fade away, but we do it for an eternal prize. So I run with purpose in every step. I am not just shadowboxing. I discipline my body like an athlete, training it to do what it should. Otherwise, I fear that after preaching to others I myself might be disqualified.**

Just as an athlete trains his body to do what it must do, we as Christ-followers must also train our bodies and renew our minds with the things of Christ. He has given us eyes to really see, ears to truly hear the Holy Spirit, and the mind of Christ to work out our salvation with fear and trembling (Matt. 13:16, Phil. 2:12).

Our hope for exiting the sex spiral is laid out specifically in Hebrews 12:1-2. The answer to living a life of forgiveness and freedom from pornography is in Jesus Christ, our Savior God. This race that you are running is one of faith, surrender, sacrifice, community, and discipline *under the grace, mercy, and forgiveness of Jesus Christ*.

CHRIST THE REDEEMER

In the opening ceremony of the 2016 Olympic games at Rio de Janeiro, there was a beautiful opening video shot of the statue, *Christ the Redeemer*. The footage from the helicopter had the statue lit up in different colors with the stadium in the background. The statue is one of the most recognizable features of any city and is regarded as one of the new seven wonders of the world.

Christ the Redeemer was created by French sculptor, Paul Landowski. An interesting note about Paul is that he won a gold medal in the art competitions in the 1928 Summer Olympics in Amsterdam for "The Boxer." The art competition was held in the Olympics from 1912 to 1952. I can't help but wonder what Paul would say about that

The Answer: Living in Freedom

beautiful opening shot of the Olympic Games in Brazil. He was a world-class athlete in his own right, and it's almost as if he consciously and deliberately put *Christ the Redeemer's* watchful eye over the stadium during those games as a reminder for us to keep our eyes fixed on Jesus as we run this beautiful race.

EPILOGUE

SO, WHERE DO YOU GO from here, my new friend? I want you to join me in this amazing and agonizing race. And I'm not *just* saying that! *I really do mean it!* I want to invite you into this race—a journey—that is one of the most thrilling, painful, and rewarding things you'll ever do. I've talked to a lot of people who say they want to start running, really running, but the reality is that very few start, and even fewer finish.

Isaiah 55:8-9 (The Voice) says, **"My intentions are not always yours, and I do not go about things as you do. My thoughts and My ways are above and beyond you, just as heaven is far from your reach here on earth."**[106]

We all need a game plan and a coach. If you would allow me, I would like to be that for you. Below are two very simple tasks to get you started.

GAME PLAN

A game plan to overcome lust consists of playing both offense and defense. Below is one play for offense and one for defense. To start your race with me as your coach, you need to follow these guidelines:

1. **Offense**: Visit DustinDaniels.org. Here, you will find not only the plan, but also daily coaching through a daily podcast called *God, Sex & You*. Sign up for the daily podcasts via iTunes.
2. **Defense**: Protect yourself and your family from pornography by signing up for Covenant Eyes (www.CovenantEyes.com). It's accountability and filtering software for all your devices. I'm an affiliate, so upon checkout, use my full name with no spaces

---

106 Ecclesia Bible Society, *The Voice*, Nashville, Thomas Nelson, 2012.

(DustinDaniels) and receive thirty days free. I've been personally using it for years and believe it's a must-have within this race.

Lastly, use *The Sex Spiral* worksheet as a timeline for the last time you acted out. You can download it for free at my website. Write in one or two words at each trigger. This will allow you to start seeing your spiral as a pattern. Once you start recognizing your own pattern, you are then able to exit the sex spiral appropriately by fleeing, praying, and confessing. If you would like to go through the workbook, find a group, or be trained as a facilitator, please visit dustindaniels.org for more information.

BIBLIOGRAPHY

Allen, D. L. *Hebrews*. Nashville: B & H Publishing Group, 2010. 574.

Alliance Defending Freedom, Blackstone Legal Fellowship Conference, 2014.

Bartolini, Peter, "Important Things About Men," (camp book for kids, 2007).

Bonhoeffer, Dieterich. *The Cost of Discipleship.* New York: MacMillian Publishers, 1959.

Carnes, Dr. Patrick. *Out of the Shadows: Understanding Sexual Addiction.* Center City: Hazelden Publishing, 1983.

Clinton, Timothy and Dr. Mark Laaser. *The Fight of Your Life: Manning Up to the Challenge of Sexual Integrity.* Shippensburg: Destiny Image Publishers, Inc., 2015.

Conklin, Kurt. "Adolescent Sexual Behavior: Demographics." AdvocatesforYouth.com. http://www.advocatesforyouth.org/publications/publications-a-z/413-adolescent-sexual-behavior-i-demographics (accessed August 9, 2017).

Countryman-Roswurm, Karen, "Why Fighting Sex Trafficking Absolutely Includes Fighting Pornography." FighttheNewDrug.org. http://fightthenewdrug.org/fighting-sex-trafficking-absolutely-includes-fighting-pornography/ (accessed May 24, 2017).

Davis, C. Truman , MD., M.S. "A Physician's View of the Crucifixion of Jesus Christ." CBN.com. http://www1.cbn.com/medical-view-of-the-crucifixion-of-jesus-christ (accessed January 2014).

DelHousaye, Darryl. "The President's Class." Class lecture, Scottsdale Bible Church, Scottsdale, AZ, 2009.

DeSilva, D. A. *Perseverance in Gratitude: A Socio-rhetorical Commentary on the Epistle "to the Hebrews."* Grand Rapids: Wm. B. Eerdmans Publishing Co., 2000.

Dustin Daniels Radio Show. "Let's Do Something About the Porn Epidemic." Episode 118. October 24, 2015.

Ecclesia Bible Society, *The Voice*, Nashville, Thomas Nelson, 2012.

Ellingworth, P., and E.A. Nida. *A Handbook on the Letter to the Hebrews.* New York: United Bible Societies, 1994. 291.

England, Dorothy Marie. *Smoke & Mirrors: The Magical World of Chemical Dependency.* Cincinnati: Forward Movement, 1995.

Ford, Nick. *Suffering & Endurance,* May 22, 2016. http://nhcc-az.com/sermons/hebrews/mediaposts/suffering-and-endurance.

Freidel, Frank and HughSidey. *The Presidents of the United States of America.* Scala Publishers, 2006.

Friends. "The One with the Free Porn." Season 4, Episode 17. Directed by Michael Lembeck. Written by Richard Goodman. National Broadcasting Company, March 26, 1998.

Gaebelein, Frank E., *The Expositor's Bible Commentary, Volume 12: Hebrews through Revelation.* Nashville: Zondervan, 1982.

Garlow, Jim, Blackstone Conference, Morning Devotion, Alliance Defending Freedom, 2013.

Bibliography

Gilkerson, Luke. "The Great Masturbation Hoax: Is Not Masturbating Unhealthy for You?" Covenanteyes.com. http://www.covenanteyes.com/2015/04/13/the-great-masturbation-hoax-is-not-masturbating-unhealthy-for-you/ (accessed July 22, 2016).

Howard, Brian Clark. "How Tornadoes Form and Why They're So Unpredictable." *National Geographic*, May 11, 2015. http://news.nationalgeographic.com/2015/05/150511-tornadoes-storms-midwest-weather-science/, July 1, 2016.

http://www.trueface.org.

https://dustindaniels.org/2017/03/01/difference-discipline-punishment.

Hughs, R. Kent. *Hebrews: An Anchor for the Soul*. Wheaton: Crossway Publishers, 2015.

Hunt, June. *Anger: Facing the Fire Within*. Self-Published, 2011.

Ledford, Heidi. "Spacesuits Optional for 'Water Bears.'" Nature.com. http://www.nature.com/news/2008/080908/full/news.2008.1087.html (September 8, 2008).

Lorence, Jordan, "The Vast Future of Marriage with Dignity," Alliance Defending Freedom: Academy Presentation. August 1, 2014, Laguna, CA.

MacArthur, John. "The Fall of Man Parts 1-2." GracetoYou.org. March 2000. https://www.gty.org/library/sermons-library/90-238/the-fall-of-man-part-1. https://www.gty.org/library/sermons-library/90-239/the-fall-of-man-part-2 (accessed October 2010).

MacArthur, John. "The Temptation of Christ." GracetoYou.org. https://www.gty.org/library/sermons-library/90-84/the-temptation-of-christ (accessed April 23, 1995).

McDaniel, Chip. *The English-Hebrew Reverse Interlinear Old Testament English Standard Version.* Lexham Press, 2009.

Miller, Jake. "15 Years Ago: Bill Clinton Historical Denial." CBS News. http://www.cbsnews.com/news/15-years-ago-bill-clintons-historic-denial/ (accessed January 26, 2013).

Morris, Chris. "Porn's Dirtiest Secret: What Everyone Gets Paid." CNBC.com. http://www.cnbc.com/2016/01/20/porns-dirtiest-secret-what-everyone-gets-paid.html (accessed June 10, 2016).

Murray, Karis Kimmel. *Grace Based Discipline: How to Be At Your Best When Your Kids Are At Their Worst.* Phoenix: Family Matters Press, 2017.

Nair, Ken. "Discovering the Mind of a Woman." Conference, Phoenix, 2016.

Nair, Ken. "Discovering the Mind of a Woman." Workshop, Thomas Nelson, Nashville, 1995.

Peterson, Eugene H. *The Message: The Bible in Contemporary Language.* Colorado Springs: NavPress, 2005.

Reyburn, W. D., and E.M. Fry. *A Handbook on Genesis.* New York: United Bible Societies, 1998. 51.

Schwandt, John. *The English Greek Reverse Interlinear New Testament English Standard Version.* Lexham Press, 2009.

Smith, Bruce: Alliance Defending Freedom—Messaging University, 2014.

Stack, Steven, Ira Wasserman, and Roger Kern. "Adult Social Bonds." *Social Science Quarterly,* 85 (2004): 75-88.

Struthers, William. *Wired for Intimacy: How Pornography Hijacks the Male Brain.* Downers Grove: Intervarsity Press, 2010.

Swindoll, Chuck. *Insights on Romans.* Grand Rapids: Zondervan, 2010.

Bibliography

The Washington Post. "What Clinton Said." WashingtonPost.com. http://www.washingtonpost.com/wp-srv/politics/special/clinton/stories/whatclintonsaid.htm (accessed May 2017).

Thrall, Bill; McNicol, Bruce; Lynch, John: *The Cure: What if God Isn't Who You Think He Is and Neither Are You?* Carol Stream: NavPress, 2011.

Thrall, Bill, Bruce McNicol, and John Lynch. *TrueFaced: Trust God and Others with Who You Really Are.* Colorado Springs: NavPress, 2004.

Tozer, A.W. *The Knowledge of the Holy.* New York: Harper One Publishers, 1961.

Turner, Mike. "Immersion Workshop Series." Workshop, Seven Places Ministries, Phoenix, January 2014.

Vincent, M. R. *Word Studies in the New Testament.* Vol. 4. New York: Charles Scribner's Sons, 1887. 537.

Weiss, Dr. Doug. *Clean: A Proven Plan for Men Committed to Sexual Integrity.* Nashville: Thomas Nelson, 2013.

DISCOGRAPHY

Seven Places, *Lonely for the Last Time.* BEC Recordings, 2003.

West, Christopher. *Your Body Tells God's Story: An Intro to St. John Paul's II,* "Theology of the Body," Audio CD. https://shop.corproject.com/cds/cd-your-body-tells-god-s-story.html.

For more information about
Dustin Daniels
&
The Sex Spiral

please visit:

www.DustinDaniels.org
www.SevenPlaces.org
@PurityPastor
www.facebook.com/PastorDustin
www.linkedin.com/in/puritypastor

For more information about
AMBASSADOR INTERNATIONAL
please visit:

www.ambassador-international.com
@AmbassadorIntl
www.facebook.com/AmbassadorIntl